Springer Wien New York

Jozef Rovenský · Burkhard F. Leeb
Howard Bird · Viera Štvrtinová · Richard Imrich
Editors

Polymyalgia Rheumatica and Giant Cell Arteritis

SpringerWienNewYork

Editors
Prof. Jozef Rovenský, MD, DSc, FRCP, Slovakia
Dr. Burkhard F. Leeb, Austria
Prof. Howard Bird, MD, FRCP, United Kingdom
Prof. Viera Štvrtinová, MD, PhD, Slovakia
Dr. Richard Imrich, Slovakia

Printed with financial support of
Roche Slovensko s.r.p., Nycomed Slovakia s.r.o. and Abbot Slovakia Ltd.

Printed in Germany
SpringerWienNewYork is part of Springer Science+Business Media
springer.at

The publisher and editor kindly wish to inform you that in some cases, despite their efforts to do so, the obtaining of copyright permissions and usage of excerpts of text is not always successful.

Photo Credits:
© Nguyen GK, Lee MW, Ginsberg J, Wragg T, Bilodeau D.: Coverphoto
© with courtesy of Assoc. Prof. MD. I. Makaiová, PhD.:
    PET scan – in Giant cell arteritis, fig. 23 and 24 (p. 91)
© all other figures with courtesy of the editors and authors

Cover Design: WMXDesign GmbH, Heidelberg, Germany
Typesetting: le-tex publishing services GmbH, Leipzig, Germany
Printing and binding: Strauss GmbH, Mörlenbach, Germany

Printed on acid-free and chlorine-free bleached paper
SPIN: 12555901

Library of Congress Control Number: 2009930748

With 27 colored figures

ISBN 978-3-211-99358-3   SpringerWienNewYork

Preface

In the present monograph, we offer current insights into polymyalgia rheumatica and giant cell arthritis. Both diseases are typical for advanced age, and their incidences increase with aging. Both diseases are a center point of interest not only for rheumatologists, gerontologists, ophthalmologists or neurologists, but also for general practitioners. Early diagnosis and rapid treatment, mainly with glucocorticoids can save one of the most precious senses-vision. Damage to other organs (heart, aorta, coronary arteries, liver, lungs, kidneys), which are supplied by the arteries affected by ischemic syndrome in the setting of giant cell arthritis, has serious consequences as well. Late diagnosis of giant cell arthritis can have fatal consequences for affected patients.

It is a matter of fact that the human population is aging. Therefore, more attention has to be paid not only to diagnosis, clinical course and treatment of rheumatic diseases in elderly, but also to their genetic, immunologic, endocrinologic, chronobiologic mechanisms, and state-of-the-art diagnostic modalities. I am convinced that the interdisciplinary research of the diseases will allow us to diagnose and treat the rheumatic diseases even faster and more effectively in the future. The monograph is a result of cooperation among five institutions; the National Institute of Rheumatic Diseases in Piestany, Slovakia; Clinical Pharmacology Unit, Chapel Allerton Hospital Leeds, United Kingdom, the Department of Rheumatology in Stockerau, Austria; the Medical School of Comenius University in Bratislava and the Institute of Experimental Endocrinology in Bratislava, Slovakia. It is my great pleasure to appreciate the Slovak Research and Development Agency (APVV) for its financial support of polymyalgia rheumatica and giant cell arthritis research (this work was supported by Science and Technology Assistance Agency under the contract. No APVT-21-032304).

On behalf of all authors,   Prof. MUDr. Jozef Rovenský, DSc. FRCP

Contents

List of Contributors

Prof. Howard Bird, MD, FRCP
Clinical Pharmacology Unit,
Chapel Allerton Hospital
Leeds, United Kingdom
E-mail: howard.bird@leedsth.nhs.uk

Ass. Prof. Stanislava Blažíčková, Ing. PhD Slovakia
National Institute of Rheumatic Diseases,
Piešťany, Slovakia
E-mail: blazickova@nurch.sk

Ass. Prof. Vladimír Bošák, Dr. PhD Slovakia
National Institute of Rheumatic Diseases,
Piešťany, Slovakia
Faculty of Health, Care and Social Work,
Trnava University,
Trnava, Slovakia
E-mail: bosak@nurch.sk

Juraj Duda, MD
County Hospital,
Michalovce, Slovakia

Richard Imrich, MD, PhD Slovakia
Center for Molecular Medicine,
Institute of Experimental Endocrinology,
Slovak Academy of Sciences,
Bratislava, Slovakia
E-mail: richard.imrich@savba.sk

Dr. Burkhard F. Leeb
1st and 2nd Department of Medicine,
Center for Rheumatology,
Lower Austria; State Hospital Stockerau,
Karl Landsteiner Institute for Clinical Rheumatology
Stockerau, Austria
E-mail: burkhard.leeb@stockerau.lknoe.at;
leeb.rheuma@aon.at

Thomas Nothnagl
1st and 2nd Department of Medicine, Centre for Rheumatology,
Lower Austria; State Hospital Stockerau;
Karl Landsteiner Institute for Clinical Rheumatology.
Stockerau, Austria
E-mail: thomas.nothnagl@stockerau.lknoe.at

Assoc. Prof. Peter Poprac MD, PhD Slovakia
National Institute of Rheumatic Diseases,
Piešťany, Slovakia
E-mail: poprac@nurch.sk

Bernhard Rintelen
1st and 2nd Department of Medicine, Centre for Rheumatology,
Lower Austria; State Hospital Stockerau;
Karl Landsteiner Institute for Clinical Rheumatology.
Stockerau, Austria
E-mail: bernhard.rintelen@stockerau.lknoe.at

Prof. Jozef Rovenský, MD, DSc, FRCP, Slovakia
National Institute of Rheumatic Diseases,
Piešťany, Slovakia
E-mail: rovensky.jozef@nurch.sk

Martin Steindl
1st and 2nd Department of Medicine, Centre for Rheumatology,
Lower Austria; State Hospital Stockerau;
Karl Landsteiner Institute for Clinical Rheumatology.
Stockerau, Austria
E-mail: martin.steindl@stockerau.lknoe.at

Svetoslav Štvrtina, MD, PhD. Slovakia
Department of Pathology
Medical Faculty Comenius University
Bratislava, Slovakia
E-mail: svetoslav.stvrtina@fmed.uniba.sk

Prof. Viera Štvrtinová, MD, PhD Slovakia
2nd Internal Clinic Medical Faculty, Comenius University,
Bratislava, Slovakia
E-mail: vierastvrtinova@centrum.cz

Alena Tuchyňová, MD, PhD Slovakia
National Institute of Rheumatic Diseases,
Piešťany, Slovakia
E-mail: tuchynova@nurch.sk

Polymyalgia Rheumatica and Giant Cell Arteritis – an overview with a focus on important factors contributing to the severity of the disease

1

Jozef Rovenský, Burkhard F. Leeb, Viera Štvrtinová,
Richard Imrich, Juraj Duda

1.1
Introduction

Polymyalgia rheumatica (PMR) and giant cell arteritis (GCA) can be regarded quite rare systemic inflammatory diseases in the general population, however, their incidence increases with increasing age, and it may be anticipated that those disorders are frequently under-recognised. To diagnose both, PMR and GCA, extensive clinical experience in rheumatology as well as in general internal medicine is mandatory. The most important prerequisite, though, is to consider the possibility of existing PMR or GCA in the respective patients. Although commonly considered typically for elderly patients (70 and above), the most recent surveys reported development of PMR and GCA also in 4th and 5th decade. Moreover, also juvenile temporary arteritis and GCA has been reported in neonates and infants with fatal consequences (1, 2).

Although PMR and GCA are commonly regarded as two clinical variations of the same disease, their clinical picture is quite different (3, 4). Whilst in PMR the musculoskeletal symptoms predominate, arterial inflammation and its consequences constitute the major features of GCA, indicating higher clinical and pathological discrepancies between the two syndromes also with respect to morbidity and mortality (5).

1.2
Clinical features

PMR as well as GCA are accompanied by a number of non-specific symptoms, such as lethargy, fatigue, fever, loss of appetite and weight, and overall weakness. William Bruce described PMR symptoms for the first time in 1888 (6) Usually, PMR shows an

1

acute onset with severe and symmetric, muscle pain in the shoulder girdle and the neck, less often in the pelvic girdle, accompanied by muscle tenderness without any swelling. Patients suffer from continuous pain often aggravated during physical inactivity or the night. However, sometimes the disease may be difficult to diagnose due to its slow and sluggishly progressing initial manifestations. Sometimes transient synovitis occurs without radiological signs of arthritis. Far too often the symptoms are thought to be primarily age-related, despite the fact that with a simple erythrocyte sedimentation rate (ESR)-testing PMR could be easily taken into consideration. Given the correct diagnosis the prognosis of PMR can be regarded excellent. Corticosteroids, the golden standard of all therapeutic measures, lead to a tremendous improvement of the affected patients in general.

GCA is a primary systemic vasculitis mainly affecting large vessels of distal aortic arch. Clinical GCA findings depend on the location and scope of vessel impairment. Hutchinson gave the first clinical description of temporal arteritis in 1890 (2) and Horton presented the histopathological findings in their relation to the clinical syndrome in 1932 (7). Later, Gilmore (8) found that this form of vasculitis may also affect other arteries and introduced the term of "giant cell arteritis". Nowadays GCA is clearly understood as a systemic disease with numerous severe and sometimes life-threatening cardiovascular complications. The variability and wide range of clinical findings and the clinical progression of the disease is presumably resulting from the heterogeneous immune and inflammatory response in the individual patient (9).

The leading clinical symptom of GCA is headache in two thirds of patients. Headache may be severe, sometimes radiating, most frequently located in the temporal area, sometimes in the occipital area, and experienced e.g. on combing hair. The temporal arteries are thickened, tender, with palpable nodules along the artery and reduced or even absent pulsation (Fig. 1). In any case of supected temporal arteritis an ultrasound examination should be performed, the typical "halo" nearly proves the diagnosis (10) Biopsy results depend on the length of the biopsy taken and the number of cuts investigated under the microscope (11). Although biopsy should be considered very important, the required treatment, however, should not be postponed due to biopsy procedure. GCA of the temporal artery does not necessarily constitute the only manifestation of the disease. Therefore, a negative biopsy of the temporal artery does not exclude GCA (12) Nevertheless, in doubtful cases a biopsy of the temporal artery may contribute to an ultimate clarification. However, it has to be pointed out that GCA of the temporal artery not necessarily constitutes the only manifestation of the disease.

1.3
Epidemiology

The annual PMR/GCA incidence is 1.7 to 7.7 per 100,000 inhabitants in elderly patients (13). The incidence of PMR increases with the age of the population. It constitutes a relatively rare disease in people below 50 years, although it may also be present in younger adults (14, 15). The younger a patient is, however, the lower the probability of PMR can be expected (16). The overall incidence in the general population totals to 20 to 50 new PMR-cases per year per 100,000 people, with a fourfold higher risk for females to become affected (17). There is evidence that the frequency of PMR-cases may be somewhat dependent on the geographical region. In Europe for example, the incidence rates are higher in the northern parts of the continent (e.g. Norway: 113 PMR cases per 100,000 inhabitants per year) in comparison to the southern parts (e.g. 13 per 100,000 per year in Italy) (18 31). In addition the frequency of newly developed PMR cases shows fluctuations over time. That is why relationships to infections, e.g. with Chlamydia or Parvovirus B19, or simply seasonal differences are in discussion (18, 19). In 15 to 20% of PMR patients the symptoms occur coexistent with biopsy proven GCA, predominantly of the temporal artery. On the contrary 40 to 60% of GCA patients have symptoms of PMR (16). PMR is more frequent than GCA. As PMR patients without cranial symptoms are very unlikely to have positive findings on temporal biopsy, this procedure is only recommended in PMR patients with cranial symptoms, such as headache or jaw claudication (20).

1.4
Laboratory findings

Laboratory changes are generally non-specific, as a hallmark the acute phase response, measured by erythrocyte sedimentation rate (ESR) or C-reactive protein (CRP) or other parameters, is usually found highly elevated, despite the fact that PMR may also exist without elevated acute phase reactants (21). Martinez-Taboada et al. (22) suggested a limit of 30 mm/hour, however Proven et al. (21) highlighted the fact that no difference in clinical findings and disease course in PMR and GCA patients with lower or higher ESR could be found, except for GCA with systemic changes, who had higher ESR values. Whether PMR with little or no elevation of acute phase reactants can be regarded a more benign disease is still in debate (21, 23). Generally mild microcytosis and thrombocytosis can be observed, while commonly the leucocytes count can be found within the normal range. Positive rheumatoid factors concentrations or elevated antinuclear antibodies are to be seen occasionally. Muscle enzymes, such as creatine-kinase or aldolase are in the normal ranges; sometimes an elevation of the alkaline phosphatase can be observed. Liver biopsy performed in a group of PMR patients with increased alkaline phosphatase activity revealed mild portal and intralobal inflammation.

Malvall et al. (24) detected increased concentrations of IgG and C3 and C4 complement components in the serum of PMR patients. Recently, the presence of IgG anticardiolipin antibodies has been reported during GCA treatment, with a decrease during glucocorticoid treatment. In addition, an increase of sIL-2R concentrations was found in patients with active PMR/GCA with a decrease after 6 months of glucocorti-

1

coid treatment. Moreover, IL-6 levels were found elevated along with the increase of the sIL-2R concentration and an increase in the number of CD8+ lymphocytes. In patients with progressing or relapsing PMR/GCA the number of CD8+ lymphocytes was found remarkably lower. Other authors reported increased factor VIII (von Wille-brand) concentrations and increased IL-2 levels in some patients (25).

IL-6 levels were recently described not only as markers for disease activity assessment, but also as prognostic markers, but did not become part of the routine laboratory program yet, as its advantage over ESR or CRP is not that pronounced considering the costs (26). All the other laboratory measures performed are rather targeted against potential differential diagnoses that to prove PMR (27, 28).

1.5
Differential diagnosis

The more unspecific the patient's symptoms are the more important become considerations about eventually existing other disorders than PMR/GCA as the reason for the patient's complaints.

Myalgia may be a symptom of several diseases. Above all late onset rheumatoid arthritis (LORA) may start with widespread myalgic complaints (29). However, arthritis, high titres of rheumatoid factors and an only partial response to low-dose glucocorticoid treatment as well as involvement of the hand and finger joints allow some distinction between LORA and PMR (29). Transient synovitis nevertheless may also be present in PMR patients, but PMR patients typically are rheumatoid factor negative. LORA (also called senile RA) typically begins as oligoarthritis with involvement of the shoulder joints. Overall manifestations of the disease are quite significant while rheumatoid factors are often negative. Sometimes the ultimate diagnosis can be clarified after a period of time. Polymyalgic syndromes may also of paraneoplastic nature (30). The recommendation to investigate PMR patients thoroughly the younger they are and the less impressive their response to corticoids is, particularly if they are male can be given as a rough rule of thumb.

PMR/GCA like symptoms may also occur with hypothyroidism, with chronic septic disorders and inflammatory myopathic disorder. Bilateral shoulder joint capsulitis can be quite easily distinguished from PMR on the basis of passive movement limitations. Such examination may also be used to differentiate between PMR and osteoarthritis of shoulder and hip joints. Also, rotator cuff impingement syndrome can be differentiated by clinical examination (painful arc). Ultrasonography, revealing shoulder joint effusion, can be regarded significantly helpful with respect to differentiate between PMR and other disorders, In addition, an elevated acute phase response as measured by ESR and CRP and joint effusion as shown by sonography or MRI is hallmarks to diagnose PMR. GCA should be considered in every patient older than 50 with newly occurred headache, temporary or permanent loss of vision, myalgia, increased ESR and fever of unknown origin. It should be emphasized that loss of vision may constitute the first manifestation of the disease, often without any prodromal symptoms. Visual disturbances have been reported more rarely in patients on corticosteroid treatment. Arteries of the head, the neck and the extremities should be examined for tenderness or possible swelling or hypertrophy, they should be investigated for murmurs along their entire length, and peripheral pulsation shall be palpated on both upper extremities and lower extremities.

Involvement of large vessels in GCA patients may result in fatal consequences. Therefore, all patients suspected to suffer from GCA should be specifically examined for possible changes in these arteries. Blood pressure has to be measured at both upper extremities, palpation for peripheral pulsation and auscultation for murmurs along large extremity vessels is highly recommended. The scope of vessel involvement can be examined using ultrasound and angiography, which may reveal smooth stenoses altered by slightly dilated sections or even occlusions. Moreover, typically bilateral localization and segmented involvement of the aorta and its branch can be visualized. Angiographic findings may guide interventions in patients not responding to conservative treatment. Negative biopsy findings do to exclude the GCA diagnosis in case of remaining clinically suspected disease. Doppler ultrasonography is a very useful and widely available method to confirm a first suspicion of vasculitis, but it has limitations especially at the large thoracic vessels, which are affected in many cases (10). Laboratory markers alone are not sufficient to evaluate disease activity. The new imaging modality PET/CT (Fig. 23, 24) provides the additional information. It allows the evaluation of disease activity and vessel morphology as well as the localization of the inflammatory process in the same session (31). Temporal arteritis may be found also in case of other vasculitis disorders, such as Wegner's granulomatosis or microscopic polyarteritis. On the other hand, inflammation of the temporal artery not necessarily occurs in all GCA patients (32).

1.6
Aetiopathogenesis

The aetiology and pathogenesis of PMR and GCA are not elucidated yet. However, considerations in this respect are focussed on environmental factors-particularly infections with Chlamydia, Mycoplasma, Parainfluenza-virus or Parvovirus B19 – and genetic ones. An association with the HLA system as well as a number of characteristic inflammatory reactions has been revealed. Cellular and humoral immune mechanisms are involved in the pathogenesis of both diseases. Some studies showed a reduction of CD8+ T-cells in both diseases. However, such a reduction has not been proven by other studies.

Increased levels of antiphospholipid antibodies have been detected in both, PMR and GCA patients. However, clinical manifestations of an antiphospholipid syndrome have been rarely reported.

The occurrence of PMR/GCA in genetically predisposed patients may also be the consequence of a number of neuroendocrine changes relating to natural aging.

Concentrations of several hormones are known to undergo changes in elderly e.g. decrease in adrenal androgen levels such as of dehydroepiandrosterone (DHEA), dehydroepiandrosterone sulphate (DHEAS) and androstenedione (ASD). Reduction of adrenal androgen levels has been inversely correlated with concentrations of pro-inflammatory cytokines such as TNF and IL-6 (33). Thus, the natural decrease of the adrenal androgens associated with an increase in the concentrations of pro-inflammatory cytokines at older age might predispose to the development of PMR and TA.

Analyses of adrenal hormones levels in patients with recent onset of PMR prior to the initiation of glucocorticoid therapy and their comparison with the levels in age- and sex-matched healthy controls showed lower DHEAS concentrations in the PMR patients (34).

Another study showed lower baseline ASD levels in untreated male patients with PMR compared with healthy controls. However, in the latter study no differences were found between basal DHEAS. Contrary to DHEAS, cortisol concentrations in patients at the time of the PMR diagnosis did however not significantly differ from those in healthy controls (35, 36). An intricate feedback system probably maintains cortisol levels within the normal range. Because of the ongoing inflammation however cortisol secretion remains insufficient (36). Also, a very good therapeutic response to the administration of exogenous glucocorticoids suggests that there might be a relative deficit of the endogenous hormones.

In another study, corticoliberin (CRH) and adrenocorticotropic hormone (ACTH) stimulation were used to evaluate the functional status of the hypothalamic-pituitary-adrenal (HPA) axis in PMR prior to the initiation of the glucocorticoid therapy. No significant difference in the response of ACTH or cortisol was found when compared to healthy controls. However, similar ACTH response resulted in a higher secretion of 17-hydroxyprogesterone, which is a cortisol precursor, and ASD during (37). In a study conducted by Pacheco et al., after low-dose ACTH challenge, higher responses of cortisol and DHEA were found in PMR patients than in control subjects (35). Changes in steroidogenesis in terms of DHEAS reduction, relative cortisol deficit accompanied by the accumulation of the precursor of the latter, could represent additional factors of the pathogenesis of PMR and GCA.

The ultimate reason for the outbreak of PMR and GCA development has not been revealed yet. It may be somewhat be similar to viral disease. A possible relation between Hepatitis B and PMR has been considered. Some studies revealed seasonal variations with respect to the onset of the disease. Mowat and Hazleman (5) stated that more PMR cases occurred in winter and summer months and less in spring and autumn. Perfetto et al. (38) consider two possible synergic mechanisms possibly involved in a season depending onset of PMR; first they found PMR/GCA peaks closely related to the epidemic peak occurrence of mycoplasma pneumoniae and parvovirus B19 infections. Second seasonal changes in the immune system making human organism more responsive to the development of various diseases including PMR.

As in rheumatoid arthritis the HLA DRB1*04 and DRB1*01 alleles are linked to an increased susceptibility to both, PMR and GCA and may also have an impact on the severity of the disease (39). Antigen recognition by T-cells in the adventitia with subsequent production of interferon-γ and activation of macrophages as well as formation of giant cells could constitute the key process for the development of GCA. Those activated macrophages produce proinflammatory cytokines such as TNF-α, IL-1 and IL-6 in the adventitia, while in the intima and media they lead to injury by producing metalloproteinases and nitric oxide. The destructive process initiated thereby and the simultaneous repair mechanisms lead ultimately to the occlusive luminal hyperplasia.

IL-6 production was found increased in serum as well as in temporal artery biopsies of PMR and GCA patients as well as a potential role of the promoter polymorphisms of IL-6 for the clinical expression of PMR and GCA (39).

1.7
Ophthalmologic manifestations in GCA patients

50% of patients were affected by significant changes in vision due to the occlusion of ocular arteries and orbital arteries Anterior ischemic optic neuropathy is often reported in GCA patients and can be regarded the primary reason for loss of vision. In the last 30 years its occurrence has significantly decreased due to the improvement in diagnosing GCA. Nevertheless, still up to 15% of the patients develop this complication. Ischemia of the anterior optic nerve is mainly reported as a result of the involvement of the posterior ciliary artery, a branch of the ophthalmic artery supplying the optic nerve's papilla. Autopsy-proven vasculitis of the posterior ciliary artery has been reported in 75% of GCA patients, usually without clinical manifestations.

Acute visual impairment often developing over night in form of blurred vision, diplopia, light scotomas, visual field narrowing or even transient or irreversible blindness (reported in less than 10% of patients) have also been reported. In more advanced cases atrophy of the optic nerve's papilla may develop. In some cases retrobulbar neuritis without any ophthalmologically noticeable changes of the optic nerve or segmental ischemia of the optic nerve papilla due to segmental optic neuritis have been reported. In such cases GCA affects the posterior ciliary artery or nutritive optic nerves. Rarely loss of vision occurs also due to an occlusion of the central artery of the retina or due to retinopathy with haemorrhage (Fig. 2a, b). Visual impairment primarily affects one eye, however, if untreated; it may turn to two-sided blindness. The occurrence of diplopia due to the involvement of the oculomotor (Fig. 3), abducens or the trochlear nerves is quite rare, and has been reported only in 2% of GCA patients. Early recognition of visual disturbances alerting potential vision impairment (temporary scotomata, phosphorescent phenomena etc.) can contribute to prevent vision loss (12, 40, 41, 42, 43, 44, 45).

Some improvement in diagnostics may be expected thanks to the use of imaging techniques, such as coloured Doppler sonography of optic vessels or fluorescent angiography enabling to determine the scope of the optic vessel impairment.

1.8
Neurovascular manifestations in GCA patients

GCA may affect the central nervous system (CNS); cranial nerves as well as peripheral nerve system. Neurological manifestations have been reported in app. 20 to 30% of the patients, caused by vasculitis of nutrition vessels. Clinical manifestations may comprise deafness, hemiparesis, depression, confusion and peripheral neuropathy (in app. 10–15% of patients) due to mononeuropathy and peripheral polyneuropathies, which are often diagnosed before the GCA diagnosis is established. Bilateral neuropathy due to GCA mainly affecting the median nerve, have been reported in up to 40% of patients. The brachial plexus may also be involved making it difficult to distinguish the disease from the oppression of C5–C6 root. Glucocorticoid treatment has been reported successful in 74% of patients, while in the other 26% of the patients no deterioration had to be noticed (46).

Aside pain in the temporal or/and occipital area, pain in the masseter muscle (masseter claudication) has been reported in 50% of patients. GCA manifestations may also include stitching pain in the tongue, loss of appetite and pain felt in mouth and pharynx due to vascular insufficiency.

Cerebrovascular impairment, in form of strokes or transitory ischemic attacks (TIAs) is only rarely observed in GCA patients; according to Nesher in 166 biopsy-proven GCA patients 6% experienced a TIA and 3% a stroke (46). It should also be mentioned that cerebral vascular accidents (CVA) have been reported primarily in elderly patients, and may be caused not by GCA, but by simultaneously progressing arteriosclerosis. Vertebrobasilar ischemia occurs more often in GCA patients (40–60%) than in patients with arteriosclerosis (15–20%). Nevertheless CVA represents one of the main reasons for they may become fatal in case of undiagnosed GCA, and late GCA diagnosis.

Ischemic accidents have been reported to occur more frequently in patients with visual disturbances and in patients with jaw claudication. It can be assumed that simultaneous application of thrombocyte-aggregation inhibitors or anticoagulants may reduce the risk for an early stroke (47), as GCA probably accelerates atherosclerotic changes (48).

Neuropsychiatry manifestations in GCA patients include disorientation, dementia, impairment of cognitive and memory functions, mood changes (depression) and psychoses. Visual hallucinations have also been reported in patients with vision impairment or loss. It should also be mentioned that GCA might constitute the basis for the development of dementia. In these patients glucocorticoid treatment may improve the patient's condition.

Audiovestibular manifestations have been reported in 7% of patients in form of monolateral or bilateral deafness, vertigo or tinnitus with a beneficial effect of glucocorticoid treatment.

1.9
Involvement of the upper and lower extremities in GCA patients

GCA-rarely affects the arteries of the upper and lower extremities. In those cases vessels distal the subclavian and brachial artery and the femoral superficial as well as the popliteal artery are involved. Claudication constitutes the leading clinical symptom.

Up to now only a few patients with histologically proven GCA in the lower extremities (LEs) have been reported. Garcia Vázques et al. (49) reports a 52 years old patient with ischemia in upper and lower extremities, more pronounced in the left leg, suffering from ischemic pain for six months without any risk factors for arteriosclerosis, such as smoking, hypertension, increased cholesterol and triglyceride levels or diabetes mellitus. Ischemic disorder of the left leg worsened up to the level III disorder, including bilateral loss of pulsation. The temporal artery was palpable, but not painful. The patient had a high sedimentation rate (112 mm/hour) and increased serum values for albumin. Angiography revealed stenosis in both subclavian arteries (30% on the right, 70% on the left side) as well as a filiform stenosis of the left superficial femoral artery and stenosis of a lower degree of the right one. GCA diagnosis has been proven by positive biopsy from both the temporal and the superficial femoral artery. Sympathectomy was performed at both sides without success, while glucocorticoid treatment, 40 mg daily dose gradually reduced to 10 mg a day, was of transient efficacy. After three months the patient relapsed and the corticosteroid dosage had to be reincreased to 30 mg a day. After two years angiographic re-examination showed significant improvement regardless of some segmental narrowing of the left femoral superficial artery and development of large collateral connections.

In 1997, Dupuy et al. (50) reported two patients with GCA of the lower extremities with an initial reduction of the walking distance down to 30 meters.

The first patient was a 61 years old woman with hypertension and without any signs of arteritis of the external carotid artery and its branches. She had a high sedimentation rate (exceeding 100 mm/hour) and C-reactive protein values (21 mg/l). Temporal biopsy was negative. She was put on nonsteroidal antirheumatic and antimalarial treatment while pain in the right foot progressed and the patient was not able to walk for more than 30 meters.

The ultrasound examination proved numerous stenoses in the femoral artery and its distal branches. (Right superficial femoral artery, popliteal and sural artery, left superficial femoral artery) Biopsy of the right superficial femoral artery showed arteritis with giant cell granulomatosis proving GCA diagnosis. Prednisone treatment (1 mg/kg body weight) and hydroxychloroquine treatment (400 mg) were successful. After one-month of treatment pain had disappeared and the walking distance could be increased. After six month of treatment the patient was able to easily walk 3 km and pulsation of the dorsalis pedis artery reoccurred. Despite of a partially narrowed superficial femoral artery, the angiographic examination showed satisfactory calibration of both tibial arteries. After a two-year treatment the patient received 5 mg prednisone/day and felt no walking limitations.

The second patient was a 65 years old woman, suffering also from Parkinson's disease with severe depression treated with levodopa, bromocriptine and tricyclic antidepressants. During one-month claudication of the lower extremities gradually worsened. The patient was also subject to dihydroergotamine treatment for persistent migraine. Despite of this treatment headache was worsening above both temporal arteries developed. The patient's sedimentation rate reached 80 mm/hour. Diagnosis of toxic dihydroergotamine effects could not be proven. Therefore, diagnostics efforts were undertaken to prove the evidence for arteritis. Ultrasound examination showed a narrowed lumen of the superficial femoral and popliteal artery on both sides, angiography revealed bilateral narrowing of the iliac, femoral and infrapopliteal arteries. Temporal artery biopsy suggested the presence of GCA as it showed clusters of lymphocyte infiltrates spread over the entire artery wall and fragmentation of the internal elastic lamina. There were neither any giant cells nor eosinophilic cells in the periadventitia. After prednisone treatment for two months (1 mg/kg/day) in combination with anticoagulants the patient's headache disappeared and she was able to easily walk without any pain for a longer distance. After one year of treatment the sedimentation rate and CRP were normal, but pulsation of the arteria dorsalis pedis did not reoccur.

Claire Le Hello et al. (51) described 8 GCA patients (6 female, 2 male), all-suffering from lower extremity claudication with acute onset. In six cases claudication represented the primary disease symptom. Angiographies revealed numerous bilateral flat-walled stenoses and thromboses. Five patients met three of the American College of Rheumatology (ACR) criteria for the diagnosis of GCA. Biopsies of the affected arteries revealed GCA in 4 patients. In one patient the CGA diagnosis was proven post mortem. In three patients GCA could not be proven histologically from biopsy of arteries of the lower extremities. However, in one of them temporal GCA could be proven. Two other patients suffered from headache and upper extremity claudication as well as angiographic signs of arteritis in the lower limbs. All the patients were subject to glucocorticoid treatment; four of them underwent vascular surgery (three bypasses and one endarterectomy). Five patients were asymptomatic after 24 to 100 months (50.6 months in average). Surgical revascularization appeared to be unsuccessful; in one patient it was even necessary to amputate the patient's extremity.

In summary the authors concluded that in case of acute onset of bilateral, fast progressing claudication with partial or complete loss of peripheral pulsation GCA should be considered. The necessity to consider GCA in cases of all unexplained peripheral arterial obliterating diseases in middle-aged and elderly patients, given the possible consequences of vascular impairment was also emphasized. The authors also refer to autopsy findings indicating that GCA, contrasting previous assumptions, cannot be considered a rare disease (52). Thus, as a consequence biopsies of the lower limb arteries in case of unclear symptomatology are recommended. Peripheral arterial obliterating disease of lower extremities may not only be caused by arteriosclerosis, but also by vasculitides, such as GCA. Laboratory findings indicating inflammation should constitute an alert for the evidence of GCA. Delayed initiation of steroid treatment may result in severe consequences for the patient including the loss of an extremity.

1.10
Other clinical manifestations

GCA as an aggressive inflammatory disease may affect arteries in all parts of the human body. Coronary arteritis may result in myocardial infarction and congestive heart failure; dissecting aortic aneurysm may result in aortic rupture (52). GCA rarely affects skin, kidneys and lungs. High sedimentation rate and CRP values can be regarded specifically relevant to consider GCA.

Case reports describing two GCA patients from eastern Slovakia also deal with the difficulties to diagnose GCA.

The first patient was a 77 years old woman suffering from seronegative rheumatoid arthritis since 1975. Patient's history revealed pain in the shoulder and pelvic girdle, long-lasting morning stiffness, weight-loss, increasing headache and one episode of acute vision loss in 1987. At that time the ESR amounted to 90 mm/hour. The patient was treated in an ophthalmologic unit. One year later, she was examined by a rheumatologist and biopsy proved temporal arteritis. Prednisone treatment (50 mg/day) was reduced at a surgical department where partial amputation of the left lower limb was performed. Histological examination proved GCA of the tibial artery. The patient died after the last amputation due to pulmonary embolism (Fig. 4a, b).

The second patient was an 83 years old woman treated at a dermatological unit due to lupus erythematosus since 1967. In 1986, the patient was for the first time examined by a rheumatologist for visual disturbances. At that time PMR with GCA and significant bilateral amaurosis was diagnosed. Clinical findings mainly comprised pain, stiffness and atrophy of the pectoral girdle muscles. The patient received glucocorticoids for a short time, which was interrupted for diarrhoea, abdominal pain and tenesmus. The patient's condition worsened progressively and she died within a short time. Autopsy revealed bilateral GCA of the temporal artery and arteritis of the renal and mesenteric arteries.

Both cases can be summarized as late diagnosed GCA, involving the temporal as well as other arteries, with insufficient glucocorticoid treatment and fatal outcome.

1.11
Prognosis of GCA and temporal arteritis

GCA is a systemic granulomatous vasculitis of unknown aetiology typically affecting the branches of carotid artery (particularly the temporal artery), but it also may affect any medium-sized or large artery. The recognition of involvement of other than cranial arteries is considered more difficult (53).

GCA in general does not significantly reduce life expectancy of the patients, if it is early diagnosed and accordingly treated (54). Save-Söderbergh at al. (13) describes the causes of death of nine GCA patients: two of them died due to myocardial infarction, another two patients due to dissecting aneurysm and five due to sudden cerebral vas-

1

cular accident. None of these patients had been treated with corticosteroids adequately. Lie (54) analysed 18 patients with extra cranial GCA and found aortic aneurysm rupture as the cause of death of 6 patients, another 6 patients died due to aortic dissection, 3 patients due to sudden cerebral vascular accident and another 3 patients due to myocardial infarction. We have described 2 patients with GCA-causing fatal aortic aneurysm dissection (55).

Temporal arteritis per se (i.e. the arteritis affecting temporal artery) cannot be regarded a life shortening disease. There is no difference regarding life expectancy between affected patients and the non-affected population, however, GCA affecting large and medium-sized vessels may develop life threatening consequences, such as aortic dissection or rupture, in myocardial infarction or cerebral vascular accident (56).

References

1. Kagata Y, Matsubara O, Ogata S et al. Infantile disseminated visceral giant cell arteritis presenting as sudden infant death. Pathol Int 1999; 49: 226–230.
2. Hutchinson J. Diseases of the arteries. On peculiar from of thrombotic arteritis of the aged which is sometimes productive of gangrene. Arch Surg 1890; 1: 323–329.
3. Evans JM, Hunder GG. Polymyalgia rheumatica and giant cell arteritis. Rheum Dis Clin North Am 2000; 26 (3): 493–515.
4. Cantini F, Niccoli L, Storri L et al. Are polymyalgia rheumatica and giant cell arteritis the same disease? Semin Arthritis Rheum 2004; 33 (5): 294–301.
5. Mowat AG, Hazleman BL. Polymyalgia rheumatica-a clinical study with particular reference to arterial disease. J Rheumatol 1984; 11 (5): 580–581.
6. Bruce W. Senile rheumatic gout. Br Med J 1888; 2: 811–813.
7. Horton BT, Magath TB, Brown GE. All under scribed from of arteritis of the temporal vessels. Mayo Clin Proc 1932; 7: 700–701.
8. Gilmore JR. Giant cell arteritis. J Pathol Bacteriol 1941; 53: 263–277.
9. Weyand CM, Goronzy JJ. Pathogenetic principles in giant cell arteritis. Int J Cardiol 2000; 75 (Suppl 1): S9–S15.
10. Blockmans D, Bley T, Schmidt W. Imaging for large-vessel vasculitis. Curr Opin Rheumatol 2009 Jan; 21 (1): 19–287.
11. Moutray TN, Williams MA, Best JL. Suspected giant cell arteritis: a study of referrals for temporal artery biopsy. Can J Ophthalmol 2008 Aug; 43 (4): 445–448.
12. Amris K, Klausen T. Oculomotor nerve paresis in patients with rheumatological disease. Possible causes and the anatomical localization of the lesion. Ugeskr Laeger 1993; 155: 320–323.
13. Säve-Söderbergh J, Malmwall BE, Andersson R et al. Giant cell arteritis as a cause of death. JAMA 1986; 255 (4): 493–496.
14. Hunder GG. Giant cell arteritis and polymyalgia rheumatica. Med Clin North Amer 1997; 81: 195–219.
15. Whittaker PE, Fitzsimmons MG. A 24-year-old man with symptoms and signs of polymyalgia rheumatica. J Fam Pract 1998; 47 (1): 67–71.
16. Salvarani C, Cantini F, Boiardi L et al. Polymyalgia rheumatica and giant cell arteritis. N Engl J Med 2002; 347: 261–271.
17. Cimmino MA, Zaccaria A. Epidemiology of polymyalgia rheumatica. Clin Exp Rheumatol 2000; 18 (4 Suppl. 20): S9–11.

18. Peris P. Polymyalgia rheumatica is not seasonal in pattern and is unrelated to parvovirus b19 infection. J Rheumatol 2003; 30 (12): 2624–2626.

19. Wagner AD, Gerard HC, Fresemann T et al. Detection of Chlamydia pneumoniae in giant cell vasculitis and correlation with the topographic arrangement of tissue-infiltrating dendritic cells. Arthritis Rheum 2000; 43 (7): 1543–1551.

20. Gabriel SE, O´Fallon MW, Achkar AA et al. The use of clinical characteristics to predict the results of temporal artery biopsy among patients with suspected giant cell arteritis. J Rheumatol 1995; 22: 93–96.

21. Proven A, Gabriel SE, O'Fallon WM et al. Polymyalgia rheumatica with low erythrocyte sedimentation rate at diagnosis. J Rheumatol 1999; 26: 1333–1337.

22. Kanik KS, Bridgeford PH, Germain BF et al. Polymyalgia rheumatica with a low erythrocyte sedimentation rate: comparison of 10 cases with 10 cases with high erythrocyte sedimentation rate. J Clin Rheumatol 1997; 3 (6): 319–323.

23. Martinez-Taboada VM, Blanco R, Armona J et al. Giant cell arteritis with erythrocyte sedimentation rate lowers than 50. Clin Rheumatol 2000; 19: 73–75.

24. Malvall BE, Bengtsson BA, Kaijser B et al. Serum levels of immunoglobulin and complement in giant-cell arteritis. J Am Med Assoc 1976; 236: 1876–1877.

25. Uddhammar AC. Von Willebrand factor in polymyalgia rheumatica and giant cell arteritis. Clin Exp Rheumatol 2000; 18 (Suppl 20): S32–S33.

26. Gonzalez-Gay MA, Rodriguez-Valverde V, Blanco R et al. Polymyalgia rheumatica without significantly increased erythrocyte sedimentation rate: a more benign syndrome. Arch Intern Med 1997; 157 (3): 317–320.

27. Kassimos D, Kirwan JR, Kyle V et al. Cytidine deaminase may be a useful marker in differentiating elderly onser rheumatoid arthritis from polymyalgia rheumatica/giant cell arteritis. Clin Exp Rheumatol 1995; 13: 641–644.

28. Chakravarty K, Pountain G, Merry P et al. A longitudinal study of anticardiolipin antibody in polymyalgia rheumatica and giant cell arteritis. J Rheumatol 1995; 22: 1694–1697.

29. Pease CT, Haugeberg G, Montague B, Hensor EM, Bhakta BB, Thomson W, Ollier WE, Morgan AW. Polymyalgia rheumatica can be distinguished from late onset rheumatoid arthritis at baseline: results of a 5-yr prospective study. Rheumatol (Oxford) 2009 Feb; 48 (2): 123–7. Epub 2008 Nov 2.

30. Keith MP, Gilliland WR. Polymyalgia rheumatica and breast cancer. J Clin Rheumatol. 2006 Aug; 12 (4): 199–200.

31. Henes JC, Müller M, Krieger J, Balletshofer B, Pfannenberg AC, Kanz L, Kötter I. [18F] FDG-PET/CT as a new and sensitive imaging method for the diagnosis of large vessel Vasculitis. Clin Exp Rheumatol 2008 May/Jun; 26 (3 Suppl 49): S47–52.

32. Jennette JCh, Falk RJ, Andrassy K et al. Nomenclature of systemic vasculitides. Proposal of an International Consensus Conference. Arthritis Rheum 1994; 17: 187–192.

33. Straub RH, Konecna L, Hrach S et al. Serum dehydroepiandrosterone (DHEA) and DHEA sulfate are negatively correlated with serum interleukin-6 (IL-6), and DHEA inhibits IL-6 secretion from mononuclear cells in man in vitro: possible link between endocrinosenescence and immunosenescence. J Clin Endocrinol Metab 1998; 83: 2012–2017.

34. Nilsson E, de la Torre B, Hedman M et al. Blood dehydroepiandrosterone sulphate (DHEAS) levels in polymyalgia rheumatica/giant cell arteritis and primary fibromyalgia. Clin Exp Rheumatol 1994; 12: 415–417.

35. Pacheco MJ, Amado JA, Lopez-Hoyos M, Blanco R et al. Hypothalamic-pituitary-adrenocortical axis function in patients with polymyalgia rheumatica and giant cell arteritis. Semin Arthritis Rheum 2003; 32: 266–267.

36. Straub RH, Gluck T, Cutolo M et al. The adrenal steroid status in relation to inflammatory cytokines (interleukin-6 and tumour necrosis factor) in polymyalgia rheumatica. Rheumatol (Oxford) 2000; 39: 624–631.

37. Cutolo M, Sulli A, Pizzorni C et al. Cortisol, dehydroepiandrosterone sulfate, and androstenedione levels in patients with polymyalgia rheumatica during twelve months of glucocorticoid therapy. Ann N Y Acad Sci 2002; 966: 91–96.

38. Perfetto F, Moggi-Pignone, Becucci A et al. Seasonal pattern in the onset of polymyalgia rheumatica. Ann Rheum Dis 2005; 64: 1662–1663.

39. Martinez-Taboda VM, Bartolome MJ, Lopez-Hoyos M et al. HLA-DRB1 allele distribution in polymyalgia rheumatica and giant cell arteritis: influence on clinical subgroups and prognosis. Semin Arthritis Rheum 2004; 34 (1): 454–464.

40. Barricks ME, Traviesa DB, Glaser JS et al. Ophthalmoplegia in cranial arteritis. Brain 1977; 100: 209–221.

41. Caselli RJ, Hunder GG, Whisnant JP. Neurologic disease in biopsy-proven giant cell (temporal) arteritis. Neurology 1988; 38: 352–359.

42. Dimant J, Grob D, Brunner NG. Ophthalmoplegia, ptosis, and miosis in temporal arteritis. Neurology 1980; 30: 1054–1058.

43. Font C, Cid MC, Coll-Vinent B et al. Clinical features in patients with permanent visual loss duc to biopsy-proven giant cell arteritis. Br J Rheumatol 1997; 36: 251–254.

44. Keltner JL. Giant-Cell Arteritis. Signs and Symptoms. Ophthalmol 1982; 89: 1101–1108.

45. Bengtsson BA, Malvall BE. The epidemiology of giant-cell arteritis including temporal arteritis and polymyalgia rheumatica: incidences of different clinical presentations and eye complications. Arthritis Rheum 1981; 24: 899–904.

46. Nesher G. Neurologic manifestations of giant cell arteritis. Clin Exp Rheumatol 2000; 18 (Suppl 20): S24–S26.

47. Gonzalez-Gay MA, Blanco R, Rodrígues-Valverde V et al. Permanent visual loss and cerebrovascular accidents in giant cell arteritis. Arthritis Rheum 1998; 41 (8): 1497–1504.

48. Štvrtinová V, Rauová L, Tuchyňová A et al. Vasculitis of the coronary arteries and atherosclerosis: random coincidence or causative relationship? In: Shoenfeld Y, Harats D, Wick G. Atherosclerosis and Autoimmunity. Amsterdam – Lausanne – New York – Oxford – Shannon – Singapore – Tokyo, Elsevier 2001; 315–327.

49. Garcia Vázques JM, Carreira JM, Seoane C et al. Superior and inferior limb ischemia in giant cell arteritis: angiography follow-up. Clin Rheumatol 1999; 18: 61–65.

50. Dupuy R, Mercié P, Neau D et al. Giant cell arteritis involving the lower limbs. Rev Rhum 1997; 64: 500–503.

51. Le Hello C, Lévesque H, Jeanton M et al. Lower limb giant cell arteritis and temporal arteritis: follow up of 8 cases. J Rheumatol 2001; 28 (6): 1407–1411.

52. Anderson R. Giant cell arteritis as a cause of death. Clin Exp Rheumatol 2000; 18 (Suppl 20): S27–S28.

53. Štvrtinová V. Primárne systémové vaskulitídy. Bratislava, SAP 1998; 210 p (in Slovak).

54. Huston KA, Hunder GG, Lie JT et al. Temporal arteritis. A 25-year epidemiologic, clinical and pathologic study. Ann Intern Med 1978; 88 (2): 162–167.

55. Lie JT. Aortic and extracranial large vessel giant cell arteritis: a review of 72 cases with histopathologic documentation. Semin Arthritis Rheum 1995; 24 (6): 422–431.

56. Štvrtina S, Rovenský J, Galbavý Š. Aneuryzma aorty ako príčina smrti pri obrovskobunkovej arteritíde. Rheumatologia 2003; 17 (3): 213–220 (in Slovak).

Polymyalgia Rheumatica, Temporal Arteritis and Occurrence of Malignant Tumors

2

Jozef Rovenský, Alena Tuchyňová

Polymyalgia rheumatica (PMR) and temporal arteritis (TA) are clinical syndromes characterized by their onset at advanced age. Little is known about the etiopathogenesis of these two nosological conditions. TA has recently been suggested to be an autoimmune syndrome that results from the immune response of the body against antigens localized in the walls of certain vessels (1). Peptides of elastin are considered to be among the presumed targets of the autoimmune reaction (2).

The clinical picture of these syndromes is variable and thus their diagnosis is rather difficult. This is also due to a lack of specific diagnostic tests, in particular to PMR. Differential diagnosis of PMR or TA requires an exclusion of several other diseases with similar symptomatology. These include primarily infections and tumors, which are more common elderly and are frequently manifested as polymyalgia-like syndrome. Naschitz et al. (3) studied the incidence of cancer in 47 patients with PMR over a period of ten years. In five of these patients, polymyalgia-like syndrome was discovered 1-3 months before malignancy was diagnosed. In all these patients, scintigraphic examination detected metastases localized in bones and joints, while the primary tumor was in the lungs (1 patient), kidneys (1 patient), colon (2 patients), and in one patient the localization of the primary tumor could not be established. An interesting observation in this series was the atypical course of the polymyalgic syndrome, which differed from classical PMR by the onset of complaints before the age of 50 years, by affecting only one typical site, asymmetrically affecting an typical localizations, by pain in the joints and by partial or delayed effect of prednisone on the relief of symptoms. The authors assumed that patients with an atypical course of PMR are at a higher risk of developing a malignancy metastasizing into bones of articulations.

On the other hand, cases of PMR and/or TA coexistence with tumor diseases have also been reported. The interval between the manifestation of PMR and TA and diagnosis of malignancy was sufficiently long for the polymyalgic syndrome not to be considered a paraneoplastic one. As early as in 1969, Mackenzie (4) described the

Table 1 Survey of published papers about the incidence of malignant tumors in patients with PMR and TA

Author (ref.)	No. of patients	Diagnosis	No. of patients with malignancy	Localization/type of tumor (s)
Kalra & Delamere (6)	Case-reports	PMR	5	Monoclonal gammopathy-acute myeloblastic leukemia, multiple myeloma, susp. Waldenström's macroglobulinemia
Montanaro & Bizzarri (7)	Case-report	PMR-like syndrome	1	Non-Hodgkin's lymphoma later transformed into acute lymphoblastic leukemia
Haga et al. (5)	185	PMR and/or TA	28	Carcinoma uteri (3), recti (5), renis (2), pancreatis (1), ovaries (1), vulvae (1), penis (1), mammae (3), ventriculi (1), testis (1), prostatae (1), coli (5), lungs (1), lymphonodorum (2)[a]
O'Keefe & Goldstraw (8)	Case-report	PMR	1	Nonsmall cell carcinoma of lungs
Tabata & Kobayashi (9)	Case-report	PMR	1	Papillary carcinoma of the thyroid gland
Kohli & Bennett (10)	Case-reports	PMR	3	Myelodysplastic syndrome
Shimamoto et al (11)	Case-report	TA	1	Acute myelogenous leukemia
Mertens et al. (12)	111	PMR and/or TA	12	Breast (1), skin (2), colon (2), stomach (2), hypernephroma (2), ovaries (1), lungs (1), Waldenström's macroglobulinemia (1)
Lie (13)	Case-report	TA	1	Adenocarcinoma of lungs

development of malignancy in one subject of a series of 76 patients with PMR. Several papers have appeared since addressing the potential association between PMR and/or TA and the incidence of malignant tumors (Table 1). Probably the most detailed study was published by Haga et al. (5) who investigated the incidence of tumor diseases in

Table 1   *(continued)*

Author (ref.)	No. of patients	Diagnosis	No. of patients with malignancy	Localization/ type of tumor (s)
Das-gupta et al (14)	Case-report	PMR	1	IgA kappa paraproteinemia
Genereau et al. (15)	Case-report	PMR	1	Urinary bladder
Gonzáles-Gay Et al. (16)	Case-report	TA	1	Chronic lymphocytic leukemia
Assi et al. (17)	Case-report	TA	1	Squamous dermatocarcinoma
Bahlas et al. (18)	149	PMR and/ or TA	4	Multiple myeloma (2), squamous cell carcinoma, carcinoid, lymphoma[a]
Liozon et al. (19)	271	TA	20	Thyroid, rectum, prostate, sigmoid colon, mediastinum, bladder, gastric, neuroendocrine, uterus, gastric, brain (astrocytoma), B cell chronic lymphocytic leukemia, refractory anemia, chronic myelomonocytic leukemia, acquired sideroblastic idiopathic anemia, chronic myelogenous leukemia.

[a] In one patient several primary localizations of the malignant tumor

185 patients with PMR and/or TA in a prospective study covering the years 1978–1983. A series of 925 subjects randomly selected from the Central Population Registry of Norway served as controls. The data obtained from the patients and from the control subjects were compared with data from the Cancer Registry of Norway. By the end of the 5-year study, malignancy was found in 27 patients (14,6%) with PMR and/or TA and in 131 subjects (14,2%) from the control group. A higher occurrence rate of malignant tumor diseases was recorded in 16 patients with histologically verified TA (24,6%). In this subgroup of patients, the rist of developing malignancy was 2,25 times higher than in the control group and 4,4 times higher compared to the other patients with PMR and TA. In 13 patients of the series, the malignancy preceded PMR and/or TA diagnosis by 4–17 years. In 14 patients of the series, PMR and/or TA were manifested first and malignancy was diagnosed in the course of three months up to seven years. In the light of the relatively long interval between the diagnosis of

malignancy and PMR and/or TA, the authors do not consider the manifestations as a paraneoplastic syndrome.

It appears that number of studies has been growing, in which authors reported the occurrence of PMR, TA and malignancies, though the majority of them were case reports. The primary localization of the malignant tumor covered a broad range. Haga et al. (5) reported predominantly tumors localised to organs, yet other authors published findings on the occurrence of leukemia (6, 11, 16), non-Hodgkin's lymphoma (7), or Waldenström's macroglobulinemia (6, 12). In our series of 26 patients (18 patients with PMR, 8 patients with TA), we did not observe any malignancies either before diagnosis of PMR or TA was established or in the course of the three-year prospective follow-up of the patients. These results are to be considered preliminary, especially with regard to the short follow-up interval from setting up the diagnosis and from the onset of treatment. We did, however, perform a research probe in a retrospective study of the clinical material of 42 patients with PMR or TA, who had been hospitalized in our Institute after 1972. Association with malignancy was detected in two patients. One of them underwent hysterectomy for rhabdomyosarcoma 9 years before PMR was diagnosed, and in the second patient breast cancer was detected one year before the appearance of PMR. Malignancy was not found in any of the patients with TA.

Pipitone and al. concluded that there is no evidence that giant cell arteritis is associated with increased prevalence of malignancies or that it may represent a paraneoplastic syndrome (19).

On the other hand Liozon et al. (20) found, that concurrent malignancy in TA is not a rare finding, observed in up to 7.4% of the cases. Solid malignancies and hematological disorders, especially myelodysplastic syndromes, may represent precipitating factors for development of TA, which are often of paraneoplastic origin. Patients with and without malignancy seem to be almost indistinguishable in terms of features and outcome of TA. Physicians should be aware of this potential association, even in typical cases.

Nevertheless, despite the above-mentioned findings, patients with giant cell arteritis and also patients with PMR may be considered at risk of developing malignancy. This assumption is supported by several factors: the higher occurrence rate of tumor diseases in subjects of advanced age, presumed derangement of some functions of the immune system in patients with TA and PMR, known coincidence of malignancies with dermatopolymyositis and vasculitis, and alterations in the immune response brought on by therapy administered. To confirm the given assumption, prospective studies need to be performed on larger series of patients. Due to the low number of patients with TA and PMR, the problem will have to be investigated in terms of international cooperation using adequate mathematical and statistical methods in evaluating the obtained results.

References

1. Weyand CM, Bartley GB. Giant cell arteritis: new concepts in pathogenesis and implications for management. Am J Ophtalmol 1997; 123: 392–395.
2. Gillot JM, Masy E, Davril M et al. Elastase derived elastin peptides: putative autoimmune targes in giant cell arteritis. J Rheumatol 1997; 24: 677–682.
3. Naschitz JE, Slobodin G, Yeshurun D et al. A polymyalgia rheumatica-like syndrome as presentation of metastatic cancer. J Clin Rheumatol 1996; 2: 305–308.
4. Mackenzie AH. The polymyalgia rheumatica syndrome. Geriatr 1969; 24: 158.
5. Haga HJ, Eide GE, Brun J et al. Cancer in association with polymyalgia rheumatica and temporal arteritis. J Rheumatol 1993; 20: 1335–1339.
6. Kalra L, Delamere JP. Lymphoreticular malignancy and monoclonal gammopathy presenting as polymyalgia rheumatica. Br J Rheumatol 1987; 26: 458–459.
7. Montanaro M, Bizzarri F. Non-Hodgkin's lymphoma and subsequent acute lymphoblastic leukemia in a patient with polymyalgia rheumatica. Br J Rheumatol 1992; 31: 277–278.
8. O'Keefe PA, Goldstraw P. Gastropleural fistula following pulmonary resection. Thorax 1993; 48: 1278–1279.
9. Tabata M, Kobayashi T. Polymyalgia rheumatica and thyroid papilary carcinoma. Int Med 1994; 33: 41–44.
10. Kohli M, Bennett RM. An association of polymyalgia rheumatica with myelodysplastic syndromes. J Rheumatol 1994; 21: 1357–1359.
11. Shimamoto Y, Matsunaga C, Suga K et al. A Human T-cell lymphotropic virus type I carrier with temporal arteritis terminating in acute myelogenous leukemia. Scand J Rheumatol 1994; 23: 151–153.
12. Mertens JCC, Willemsen G, Van Saase JLCM et al. Polymyalgia rheumatica and temporal arteritis: a retrospective study of 111 patients. Clin Rheumatol 1995; 14: 650–655.
13. Lie JT. Simultaneous clinical manifestations of malignancy and giant cell temporal arteritis in a young woman. J Rheumatol 1995; 23: 367–369.
14. Das-gupta E, Bandyopadhyay P, Kok Shun JL. Polymyalgia rheumatica, temporal arteritis and malignancy. Postgrad J Med 1996; 72: 317–318.
15. Genereau T, Koeger AC, Chaibi P, Bourgeois P. Polymyalgia rheumatica with temporal arteritis following intravesical Calmette-Guérin bacillus immunotherapy for bladder cancer. Clin Exp Rheumatol 1996; 1: 110.
16. Gonzáles-Gay MA, Blanco R, Gonzáles-López MA. Simultaneous presentation of giant cell arteritis and chronic lymphocytic leukemia. J Rheumatol 1997; 24: 407–408.
17. Assi A, Nischal KK, Uddin J, Thyveetil MD. Giant cell arteritis masquerading as squamous cell carcinoma of the skin. Br J Rheumatol 1997; 36: 1023–1025.
18. Bahlas S, Ramos-Remus C, Davis P. Clinical outcome of 149 patients with polymyalgia rheumatica and giant cell arteiritis. J Rheumatol 1998; 25: 99–104.
19. Pipitone N, Boiardi L, Bajocchi G, Salvarani C. Long-term outcome of giant cell arteritis. Clin Exp Rheumatol 2006; 24 (Suppl. 41): 65–70.
20. Liozon E, Loustaud V, Fauchais AL et al. Concurrent Temporal (Giant Cell) Arteritis and Malignancy: Report of 20 patients with review of the literature. J Rheumatol 2006; 33 (8), 1606–1614.

Coronary involvement and atherosclerosis in Giant Cell Arteritis

3

Viera Štvrtinová, Jozef Rovenský, Alena Tuchyňová

Myocardial ischemia and its extreme consequence, acute myocardial infarction are generally accepted to be a result of transient or prolonged discrepancy between real myocardial needs for oxygen and the actual blood flow through the coronary arteries into the cardiac muscle. There may be a variety of reasons for insufficient blood supply into the coronary arteries. In industrialized countries, coronary heart disease (CHD) is caused by atherosclerosis in more than 90% of the cases: it should be borne in mind however that there is a wide range of other pathological processes that eventually may result in myocardial infarction (1) (Table 2).

Table 2   Causes of myocardial ischemia (adjusted according to Cheitlin and Virmani)

1. **Coronary atherosclerosis**
2. **Other diseases involving coronary arteries**
– arteritis (occurring in the framework of primary and secondary vasculitis)
– metabolic disease (mucopolysaccharidoses, homocysteinuria, Fabry's disease, amyloidosis, pseudoxanthoma elasticum etc.)
– compression of the coronary artery from the outside (e.g. by tumor)
3. **Coronary artery aneurysms**
4. **Coronary artery thrombosis**
5. **Coronary artery spasms**
6. **Coronary artery embolism**
7. **Congenital abnormalities of coronary arteries**
8. **Injuries and dissections**
9. **Disproportion between oxygen needs and supply** (aortic stenosis aortic insufficiency, thyreotoxicocis, pheochromocytoma, etc.)
10. **Syndrome X** (small vessel disease)

3

Inflammatory affection of the coronary arteries may present a life-threatening condition and the uderlying reason for CHD in all age groups. Since the epicardial coronary arteries are not easily accessible to biopsy, as well as the pathogenesis and classification of various forms of vasculitis are rather confusing, diseases involving the coronary arteries are rarely diagnosed correctly during the lifetime of the patients. However, a correct and timely diagnosis has become vitally important not only for the necessity to aggressively manage some "malignant" forms of vasculitis by immunosuppressive therapy, but also because of the needless administration of such therapy may lead to serious complications and adverse effects. It is therefore rather crucial to make an early distinction between vasculitis, i. e. inflammatory condition of the coronary artery, and atherosclerotic alterations since the management of the two conditions would be approached differently (2).

On the other hand, underlying vasculitis may enhance atherogenesis and the development of atherothrombosis. Smoking, hyperlipidemia, hypertension and diabetes mellitus as the major risk factors for the development and progression of atherosclerosis cannot explain atherosclerosis in many patients. A number of additional risk factors, which might be affected by systemic or local inflammation, have been identified during recent years – including elevated levels of homocysteine, lipoprotein (a), oxidative or enzymatic modifications of lipoproteins, estrogen deficiency, hypercoagulability and last but not least infection. Increasing evidence suggests that atherosclerosis is a chronic inflammatory disease developing in response to certain specific injury of vascular wall. Vascular wall inflammation plays a significant role in both the development of atherosclerosis and during the later stages when inflammation is considered to be the reason for the instability of the atherosclerotic plaque. Macrophages, endothelial cells, smooth muscle cells and activated lymphocytes are the principal constituents of the atherosclerotic plaque. Similar to an inflammatory process there is an interaction between effector cells of the immune response and the production of soluble mediators (cytokines, chemokines and soluble adhesion molecules). Markers of systemic inflammation such as C-reactive protein or serum amyloid A appear to predict cardiovascular events in healthy men and aspirin seems to significantly reduce the risk of myocardial infarction in individuals with high CRP levels only. Statins in addition to reduction of blood lipid levels modify endothelial function, inflammatory responses, plaque stability, and thrombus formation and thus reduces the risk of cardiovascular complications.

For the human vasculitides as well as atherosclerosis both autoimmune and infectious causes have been proposed (3). The primary symptoms of many vasculitides resemble those of infectious diseases and moreover, vasculitis is a well-documented manifestation of infection by some known microbial agent. In addition, in chronic or "extinguished" syphilitic arteritis, alterations of the intima resemble atherosclerotic changes, and atherosclerotic lesions may frequently by layer onto old syphilitic lesions. The organisms implicated (*Chlamydia pneumoniae, Helicobacter pylori)* as well as herpes viruses (mainly cytomegalovirus) are ubiquitous and this has raised question whether they may in some patients enhance inflammation in atherosclerosis whereas in others, e.g. in patients with altered immune function, lead to systemic vasculitis. It however remains unclear whether infectious agents act in the develop-

Table 3 The group of our patients with giant cell arteritis

Patient	Gender	Year of birth	Age at the onset	Histology	Stroke	IM	PMR
1	male	1926	74	+	0	0	0
2	female	1919	76	+	0	0	0
3	female	1931	66	+	0	+	0
4	female	1925	73	+	0	0	0
5	male	1941	51	+	0	0	0
6	female	1921	75	+	0	0	0
7	female	1924	72	+	0	0	0
8	female	1939	54	+	0	0	0
9	male	1926	70	+	0	0	0
10	female	1917	81	+	0	0	0
11	female	1919	55	+	0	0	0 PAOD
12	female	1924	73	+	0	+	0
13	female	1914	84	+	0	0	0
14	male	1926	64	not done	+	0	1
15	male	1923	77	+	+	+	0
16	female	1936	56	not done	0	0	1
17	female	1912	61	+	0	++	1
18	female	1926	58	+	0	0	1
19	female	1920	55	+	0	0	1
20	female	1912	64	+	0	0	1
21	male	1919	67	+	0	0	1
22	male	1903	72	+	0	0	1
23	male	1903	75	+	0	0	1
IM: myocardial infarction, PMR: polymyalgia rheumatica, PAOD: peripheral arterial obliterative disease of the lower extremities							

ment of atherosclerotic lesions as a cause or as a cofactor or whether they are present just as an innocent commensal.

The involvement of the coronary arteries in GCA patients is rarely recognized, though deaths have been reported due to acute myocardial infarction (4). Freddo et al. (5) suggest that myocardial infarction may be a more common early complication of temporal arteritis than appreciated and can occur despite administration of high-dose corticosteroid therapy.

In our group of 23 patients (15 females and 8 males) with the diagnosis of GCA (Table 3) four patients developed myocardial infarction, 2 patients suffered stroke and 1 patient both myocardial infarction and stroke. One female patient developed peripheral arterial obliterative disease of the lower extremities (6).

In view of the high age of patients with GCA their coronary heart disease may be assumed to atherosclerotic alterations of the coronary arteries. However, vasculitis can set in the vascular wall already damaged by the atherosclerotic process and the inflammatory response can be triggered by so far unknown mechanism. Moreover, when healed up, giant cell arteritis may only hardly be distinguished from atherosclerosis,

3

and some pathologists claim that atherosclerosis and giant cell arteritis may be based on a common pathological process. This could explain why GCA develops mainly in elderly patients. A multicentric prospective study involving 400 patients with the diagnosis of GCA or PMR identified smoking and previous arterial disease as a risk factor for the development of the GCA in women. Interestingly, patients with GCA had lower cholesterol levels at the time of the diagnosis compared to a control group of healthy volunteers: the inflammatory process may however have influenced the cholesterol levels.

References

1.   Cheitlin MD, Virmani R. Myocardial infarction in the absence of coronary atherosclerotic disease. In: R.Virmani, M.B.Forman, editors. Nonatherosclerotic ischemic heart disease. New York: Raven Press 1989; 1–30.
2.   Herve F, Choussy V, Janvresse A et al. Aortic involvement in giant cell arteritis. A prospective follow up of 11 patients using computed tomography. Rev Med Interne 2006; 27 (3): 196–202.
3.   Lee SJ, Kavanaugh A. Autoimmunity, vasculitis and autoantibodies. J Allergy Clin Immunol 2006; 117 (2): S445–S450.
4.   Karger B, Fechner G. Sudden death due to giant cell coronary arteritis. Int J Legal Med 2006; 120 (6): 377–379.
5.   Freddo T, Price M, Kase C, Goldstein MP. Myocardial infarction and coronary artery involvement in giant cell arteritis. Optom Vis Sci 1999; 76: 14–18.
6.   Štvrtinová V, Rauová Ľ, Tuchyňová A, Rovenský J. Vasculitis of the Coronary Arteries and Atherosclerosis: Random Coincidence or Causative Relationship? In: Y. Shoenfeld, D. Harats, G. Wick, editors. Atherosclerosis and Autoimmunity. Amsterdam – Lausanne – New York – Oxford – Shannon – Singapore – Tokyo: Elsevier Science 2001; 315–327.

T cells and their role in Polymyalgia Rheumatica and Giant Cell Arteritis

4

Stanislava Blažíčková, Jozef Rovenský

Giant cell arteritis (GCA) and polymyalgia reumatica (PMR) are two closely related syndromes affecting elderly people. Dramatic changes with age are characteristic for immune system. Immunosenescence has been recognized as component autoimmunity. General experience says that with age the capacity to generate protective immune response declines whereas reactivity to autoantigens increases.

GCA and PMR is an inflammatory condition of unknown aetiology. The pathological finding in GCA is granulomatous infiltrates in the wall and medium sizes arteries (1). Immunohistochemical studies have shown that CD4+T lymphocytes and monocytes/macrophages are the dominant cell populations in the infiltrates. Weyand et al. (2) provided evidence recently for clonal expansion of CD4+ T cells in vascular lesions. A minority of tissue-infiltrating T cells was present in multiple copies, and CD4+ T cells with identical T cell receptor β chains were isolated from distinct vasculitic foci. Clonal expansion of CD4+ T cells and restriction in the polymorphism of antigen-driven HLA-DR molecules support the model that GCA is an antigen- driven disease in the wall of medium sizes arteries. Wagner et al. (3) have searched for CD4+ interferon γ (IFN-γ)+ T cells in temporal artery specimens. Interestingly, only 2 to 4% of all T cells in the arterial wall have the capability of releasing IFN-γ. Although this observation raises the point that only small subsets of T cells may be disease relevant, these frequencies are compatible with the local activation of antigen-specific T cells. Indeed, CD4+ IFN-γ+ T cells in GCA lesions display several features that identify them as the T cells recently stimulated by specific antigen. Clonal expansion T cells were not detected in peripheral blood, indicating that there is accumulation of such T cells in tissue.

Besides T lymphocytes, macrophages are the second components of the vascular lesions. Their role in the inflammatory events in the arterial wall is unclear. Several functions of macrophages could be of significance in initiating and maintaining the tissue infiltrate in GCA. Data of Wagner et al. (4) support the view that an additional

4

component of systemic monocytes activation exists. It is possible that the activation of circulating monocytes results from an immune response to the same antigen in other tissues than the temporal artery, e.g. lymph nodes and bone marrow. Function activities of T cells and macrophages that accumulate in the arterial wall have been determined by analysing the transcription of cytokines and monokines in extract from temporal artery biopsies. Compared with noninflamed temporal arteries, inflamed specimens contain the T cell products IFN-γ and interleukin –2 (IL-2) and the CD68[+] macrophage products IL-1 beta, IL-6 and transforming growth factor β (TGF-β). TGF-β was most abundantly found and was produced in conjunction with, but also in the absence of IL-1β and IL-6. Comparison of circulating and tissue-infiltrating CD68[+] cells in GCA patients revealed two interesting finding. Circulating CD68[+] cells were activated in high frequency and the composition of the peripheral and tissue compartments was clearly distinct, raising the possibility of selective recruitment into the vascular lesions. The presence of similar frequencies of CD68[+] IL-6[+] cells in PMR and GCA patients demonstrates that the activation of peripheral monocytes does not require the vasculitic component of the disease. Whether the availability of IL-6 and IL-1β producing monocytes in blood is prerequisite preceding the formation of the vasculitic lesions is possible but unanswered (4). In patients with PMR, cytokine mRNA can be detected in temporal artery tissue specimens despite the lack of microscopic evidence of tissue infiltrating cells (2). The low number of tissue infiltrating macrophage and sensitivity of the polymerase chain reaction may explain the finding of the low frequency of IL-6 in tissue of PMR patients. In contrast to macrophage activation, the T cell response appears to be quantitatively, but also qualitatively, different on the two diseases. Although patients with GCA and those PMR did not differ in their in situ production of IL-2, the presence of INF-γ sequences was significantly different. IFN-γ mRNA is more easily detected in active T cells than is IL-2 mRNA, indicating that the also absence of INF-γ in the tissue of PMR patients is of biological significance and is not a result of insufficient sensitivity. IFN-γ is crucial for macrophage activation and for granuloma formation. Thus the production of IFN-γ may be essential for the development of vasculitis. Patients with PMR may lack an important amplification mechanism in their local immune response in the vasculitic lesion (2). Tissue synthesis of tumour necrosis α and granulocyte-macrophage colony-stimulating factor has not been informative in distinguishing normal and inflamed temporal arteries. Clinical experience has shown that it is often difficult to document the presence or absence of vasculitis in patients with PMR. Weyand et al. (2) had shown that PMR and GCA share multiple pathogenic features in addition to similarities in the clinical presentation. Both disease have in common an association with selected HLA-DRB1 alleles in particular the HLA-DRB1*04 alleles (5, 6). Patients with PMR and GCA have highly elevated levels of serum IL-6. After initiating corticosteroid therapy IL-6 concentration abruptly return to normal and remain suppressed as long steroid therapy is continued.

B cells are extremely rare in the vascular lesions, which is consistent with the lack of antibody production and of immune complex deposition or hypergammaglobulinemia in GCA. Even patients with GCA and concomitant chronic lymphatic leukaemia, in which B cells are typically found to infiltrate diffusely into tissue, the temporal arterial lesions contain very few B cells, raising the possibility that vasculitic infiltrates are a disfavoured environment for B cells (7).

Accumulating evidence indicates that GCA represents the consequences of a local immune to a disease – inducing antigen, and it is considered the best example of T cell mediated vasculitis (8). In the vasculitic lesions, which also express activation surface markers, undergo clonal proliferation in the inflammatory lesions of temporal artery.

TCR repertoire has been examined in patients with PMR and GCA in three recent studies (9, 10, 11). In both of them patients with PMR and GCA carried multiple expanded T cell populations, especially within the CD8$^+$ T cells subset. Although a significant number of these selected clonotypes decreased in size with high dose steroid treatment, all of them persisted despite successful control of the disease with treatment (12). Because GCA and PMR display strict age dependence, it can be hypothesised that age-related change in the TCR repertoire render individuals susceptible to the disease. To address this hypothesis Martinez-Taboada et al. (9) have compared a cohort of 18 patients with GCA or PMR with 9 age-matched controls. The frequency of clonal expansion was not different in two cohorts. Sequence analysis of the CD8 clonotypes indicated a distinct Jβ gene segment usage in the patients compared with normal control. In individual patients preferential rearrangement of selected Jβ gene elements was found, raising the possibility that a Jβ-specific mechanism was involved in driving the clonal proliferation of CD8$^+$ T cells in GCA and PMR. Because oligoclonality in the CD8 subset persisted despite successful treatment of the disease, Weyand et al. (13) have proposed that such clonotypes are not directly involved in the disease process. However, the preexisting T cell repertoire might modulate an individual's risk of generating a pathologic T cells.

In contrast with studies (9, 14, 15) Lopez-Hoyos et al. (11) did not find a clear correlation between T cell expansions and disease activity. The analysed TCR repertoire of circulating T lymphocytes with nine BV-specific monoclonal antibodies, which account for about 40–50% of the total cell repertoire. Patients with active disease had higher percentage of CD4$^+$/BV3$^+$ T cells than healthy control. However, there were no differences between patients and controls in any of the TCR BV families of the CD8$^+$ subsets. A new analysis carried out in patients with PMR and GCA six months after steroid therapy, when they were asymptomatic, showed no significant changes in the distribution of the TCR BV expansions, suggesting that these expanded populations probably are not directly involved in the disease process (11).

However, much less is known about the role circulating T cells in patients with GCA and PMR. The open is question about of number of circulating T cells and other subtypes in patients with PMR and GCA. When PMR/GCA patients non treatment were compared with controls, Macchioni et al. (16) observed a significant reduction in the absolute number and relative percentage of CD4$^-$ CD8$^+$, CD3$^-$ HLA-DR$^+$ and CD3$^+$ CD16$^+$ and or CD56$^+$ cells. CD4/CD8 cell ratio was significantly higher in PMR/GCA patients compared to controls. No significant differences in the relative percentage and absolute number of the other lymphocytes subsets (CD5$^+$CD20$^-$, CD5$^+$CD20$^+$, CD3$^+$HLA-DR$^+$, CD4$^+$CD8$^-$, CD8$^-$CD57$^+$, CD8$^+$CD57$^+$, CD3$^-$CD56$^+$) considered were observed when compared to controls. Some reports have described a decreased percentage of circulating CD8$^+$ cells before treatment and persisting for some months

4

during corticosteroid therapy. The CD8$^+$ lymphocytes are heterogeneous in subpheno-types and functions. CD8$^+$ cells include T cells, which express high-density CD8$^+$ (CD8$^{bright+}$) and not T cells with natural killer (NK) activity, which express low-density CD8$^+$ (CD8^{dim+}). Bioardi et al. (17) reported the phenotypic characterisation of CD8$^+$ subsets of patients with active PMR. They found that the percentage CD8$^{bright+}$ was significantly lower in patients with active PMR (44%) compared to controls matched for age and sex, both subsets of CD8$^{bright+}$CD57$^+$ and CD8$^+$ CD57$^-$ were significantly reduced. The absolute of CD8$^{bright+}$ cells returned to the normal range after 3 months of steroid therapy. However, the absolute numbers of these subsets at the end follow-up (2 yr.) were lower to those of normal control. The changes in the absolute number of CD8$^{bright+}$CD57$^+$ and CD8$^{bright+}$CD57$^-$ cells during the follow-up paralleled the varia-tions of CD8$^{brigth+}$ cells. The percentage of CD8$^{bright+}$ increased significantly after 1 yr. of steroid therapy compared to baseline values, but they remained significantly lower compared to controls for the entire 2 yr. follow-up period. The percentage of CD8$^{bright+}$CD57$^-$ cells increased significantly after 6 months of therapy, even if the first and second year values were significantly lower compared to the control. GCA before treatment, Andersson et al. (18) found normal numbers of CD8$^+$ and CD4$^+$ cells and Banks et al. (19), documented normal ratios of helper to supressor cell. Other studies in patients with PMR and GCA have found a decreased percentage of CD8$^+$ cells (20, 21, 22, 23), although Dasgupta et al. (21) and Elling et al. (20) also reported reduced abso-lute number of CD8$^+$ cells. Significantly reduced percentages and number of CD8$^+$ cells have been found in 40% to 80% of patients with PMR and GCA (20, 24, 25, 26). All of the studies apart from the negative study by Andersson (18) used mononuclear cells separated on Ficoll-Hypaque density gradient. This method selectively decreases the CD8$^+$ subsets than the whole blood analysis. This artefact would not necessarily affect samples form controls and patients to the same extent, so could distort the results. Patient CD8$^+$ cells might have intrinsic differences form control cells affecting their migration on a density gradient and might well also have differences due to a delay in processing compared with control cells. A marked decrease in the percentage of CD8$^+$ and CD4$^+$ cells has been shown in blood stored for 24 hours when the Ficoll-Hypaque method used, but not with whole blood lysis method (27). Furthermore, a delay of more than six hours before processing blood samples results in a considerable decrease in the absolute number of lymphocytes counted by automated haematology counters (28). Such a delay might occur more often with patient sample than control samples, particularly in multicentre studies where patient blood samples may be transported from other hospitals for analysis.

Although in fact other biological variables may be of major importance, it has been suggested that two populations of patients with PMR/GCA are present. A persistently reduced percentage of CD8$^+$ after six months of treatment has been correlated to more severe disease (25). Reduced levels of CD8$^+$ cells and concomitantly reduced concen-trations of CD8$^+$ cells have also been found in first degree relatives of patients with GCA, indicating it to be a hereditary characteristic (29).

Corrigall et al. (30) on the basis of their results showed that patients presenting with a clinical picture of PMR can be divided into 2 groups on the basis of their pretreatment % CD8$^+$ T cells: one group with low CD8$^+$ T cells, have true PMR on follow-up while the

2nd, with normal % CD8$^+$, go to develop other diseases on follow-up, the commonest one being seronegative rheumatoid arthritis. A further group of patients identified as having normal values for % CD8$^+$ were later diagnostic as having various malignancies.

There is an evidence for associated changes in the distribution of T cell subsets in the circulating T cells compartment (31). The significant findings as well as an inverse relation of naive and memory CD4$^+$ T cells, normal expression of surface marker indicating activation of T cells, the severe depletion of CD8$^+$CD28$^+$ circulating T cells may contribute to the development of disease in two different ways. Firstly, it may reflect a possible infectious agent, especially a viral infection, as responsible for these syndromes. An increasing amount of epidemiological, clinical and laboratory evidence support this hypothesis (32). Secondly, and not mutually exclusive from the first hypothesis, the loss expression of CD28 with ageing may contribute to state of immunodeficiency that may make a susceptible person prone to develop a disease (33).

References

1.   Huston KA, Hunder GC, Lie JT et al. Temporal arteritis – a 25-years epidemiological, clinical, and pathologic study. Ann Intern Med 1978; 88: 162–167.
2.   Weyand CM, Hicok CK, Hunder GG, Goronzy JJ. Tissue Cytokine Patterns in Patients with Polymyalgia Rheumatica and Giant Cell Arteritis. Ann Intern Med 1994; 121: 484–491.
3.   Wagner DA, Bjornsson J, Bartley GB et al. Interferon gamma producing T cells in giant cell vasculitis represent a minority of tissue infiltrating cells and are located distant from the site of pathology. Am J Pathol 1996; 148: 1925–1933.
4.   Wagner DA, Goronzy JJ, Weyand CM. Functional Profile of Tissue-infiltrating and Circulating CD68+ Cells in Giant Cells Arteritis. J Clin Invest 1994; 94: 1134–1140.
5.   Weyand CM, Hicok CK, Hunder GG, Goronzy JJ. The HLA-DRB1 locus as a genetic component in giant cell arteritis. Mapping of a disease-linked sequence motif to the antigen-binding site of the HLA-DR molecule. J Clin Invest 1992; 90: 2355–2361.
6.   Weyand CM, Hunder NN, Hicok CK et al. HLA-DRB1 alleles in polymyalgia rheumatica, giant cell arteritis and rheumatoid arthritis. Arthritis Rheum 1993; 36: 1286–1294.
7.   Martinez-Taboada VM, Brack A, Hunder GG et al. The Inflammatory Infiltrate in Giant Cell Arteritis Selected Against B Lymphocytes. J Rheumatol 1996; 23: 1011–101.
8.   Weyand CM, Goronzy JJ. Giant cell arteritis as an antigen driven disease. Rheum Dis Clin North Am 1995; 21: 1027–1039.
9.   Martinez–Taboada VM, Goronzy JJ, Weyand CM. Clonally expanded CD8 T cells in patients with polymyalgia rheumatica and giant cell arteritis. Clin Immunol Immunopathol 1996; 79: 263–270.
10. Grunewald J, Andersson R, Rydberg L et al. CD4+ and CD8+ T cell expansions using TCR V and J gene segments at the onset of giant cell arteritis. Arthritis Rheum 1994; 37: 1221–1227.
11. Lopez-Hoyos M, Bartolome-Pacheco MJ, Blanco R et al. Selective T cell receptor decrease in peripheral blood T lymphocytes of patients with polymyalgia rheumatica and giant cell arteritis. Ann Rheum Dis 2004; 63: 54–60.
12. Martinez-Taboada VM, Hunder GG, Weyand CM, Goronzy JJ. Steroid responsiveness of clonal CD8 populations in giant cell arteritis. Arthritis Rheum 1995; 38 (Suppl): 189.
13. Weyand CM, Goronzy JJ. Multisystem interactions in the pathogenesis of vasculitis. Cur Opin Rheumatol 1997; 9: 3–11.

14. Nityanand S, Giscombe R, Srivastava S et al. A bias in the alpha beta T cell receptor gene usage in Takayasu´s arteritis. Clin Exp Immunol 1997; 107: 261–268.

15. Esin S, Gul A, Hodara V et al. Peripheral blood T cells expression in patients with Bechcets disease. Clin Exp Immunol 1997; 107: 520–527.

16. Macchioni P, Boiardi L, Salvarani C et al. Lymphocyte subpopulations analysis in peripheral blood in polymyalgia rheumatica/giant cell arteritis. Br J Rheumatol 1993; 32: 666–670.

17. Boiardi L, Salvarani C, Macchioni P et al. CD8+ lymphocyte subsets in active polymyalgia: comparison with elderly-onset and adult rheumatoid arthritis and influence of prednisone therapy. Br J Rheumatol 1996; 35: 642–648.

18. Andersson R, Hansson GK, Soderstrom T et al. HLA-DR expression in the vascular lesion and circulating T-lymphocytes of patients with giant cell arteritis. Clin Exp Immunol 1988; 73: 82–87.

19. Banks PM, Cohen MD, Ginsburg WW, Hunder GG. Immunohistologic and cytochemical studies of temporal arteritis. Arthritis Rheum 1983; 26: 1201–1207.

20. Elling P, Olsson A, Elling H. CD8+ T lymphocyte subset in giant cell arteritis and related disorders. J Rheumatol 1990; 17: 225–227.

21. Dasgupta B, Duke O, Timme AM et al. Selective depletion and activation of CD8+ lymphocytes form peripheral blood of patients with polymyalgia rheumatica and giant cell arteritis. Ann Rheum Dis 1989; 48: 307–311.

22. Elling P, Olsson A, Elling H. A reduced CD8+ lymphocytes subset distinguishes patients with polymyalgia rheumatica and temporal arteritis form patients with other diseases. Clin Exp Rheumatol 1998; 16: 155–160.

23. Chelazzi G, Broggini M. Abnormalities of peripheral blood lymphocytes subsets in polymyalgia rheumatica. Clin Exp Rheumatol 1984; 2: 333–1136.

24. Blažíčková S, Tuchyňová A, Rovenský J, Poprac P. Circulating T cell subpopulations in polymyalgia rheumatica. Zdrav vestn 2006; 75 (Suppl 1): 1–8.

25. Salvarani C, Boiardi L, Macchioni P et al. Role of peripheral CD8 lymphocytes and soluble IL-2 receptor in predicting the duration of corticosteroid treatment in polymyalgia rheumatica and giant cell arteritis. Ann Rheum Dis 1995; 54: 640–644.

26. Arnold M, Corrigall V, Panayi GS. The sensitivity and specificity of reduced CD8 lymphocyte levels in diagnostic of polymyalgia rheumatica/giant cell arteritis. Clin Exp Rheumatol 1993; 11 (6): 62–634.

27. Ashmore LM, Shopp GM, Edward BS. Lymphocytes subsets analysis by flow cytometry. Comparison of three different staining techniques and effect of blood storage. J Immunol Methods 1989; 118: 209–215.

28. Bird AG. Monitoring of lymphocytes subpopulation changes in the assessment of HIV infection (editorial review). Genitourin Med 1990; 66: 133–137.

29. Johansen MK, Elling P, Olsson AT, Elling H. A genetic approach to the pathogenesis of giant cell arteritis. Depletion of CD8+T cells in first-degree relatives of patients with polymyalgia rheumatica and arteritis temporalis. Clin Exp Rheumatol 1995; 13: 745–747.

30. Corrigall VM, Dolan AL, Panay GS. The value of percentage of CD8+ T lymphocyte levels in distinguishing polymyalgia rheumatica from early rheumatoid arthritis. J Rheumatol 1995; 22: 1020–1024.

31. Martinez-Taboada VM, Bartolome-Pacheco MJ, Amado JA et al. Changes in peripheral blood lymphocyte subsets in elderly subjects are associated with an impaired function of the hypophalamic-pituitary-adrenal axis. Mech Ageing Dev 2002; 126: 1477–1486.

32. Levine SM, Helmann DB. Giant cell arteritis. Curr Opin Rheumatol 2001; 14: 3–10.

33. Effros RB. Loss CD28 expression on lymphocytes: a marker of replicative senescence. Dev Comp Immunol 1997; 21: 471–478.

Jozef Rovenský, Richard Imrich

Cytokines play an important role in the regulation of immune responses. Markedly elevated interleukin 6 (IL-6) and IL-1 receptor antagonist concentrations were found at the time of PMR diagnosis, thus prior to start of glucocorticoid therapy. On the other hand, systemic concentrations of other antiinflammatory cytokines, such as tumor necrosis factor (TNF) and IL-1 beta were comparable with those measured in healthy controls (1).

Biopsy samples of temporal arteries showed mononuclear cell, T-cell and macrophage infiltration in the vascular wall, and disturbed lamina elastica of the temporal artery. IgG, IgM and IgA, complement and fibrinogen deposits were identified in the lesions. Moreover, enhanced IL-1 beta and interferon (IFN) gamma production and slightly reduced production of TNF were identified (2). IFN gamma seems to be an important factor, which modulates hyperplasia of the intima in the inflammation-affected vessels (3).

Systemic concentrations of IL-6 are elevated in GCA. IL-6 in the media of vessels is mainly produced by macrophages, whereas it is also produced by fibroblasts in the intima. Expression of the gene for IL-6 was not observed in endothelial cells or giant cells. As a result of glucocorticoid therapy, systemic concentrations of IL-6 decrease. IL-6 production in the involved arteries may thus contribute to general symptoms of GCA (4). In GCA and PMR patients, expression of IL-6 and IL-1 beta was observed in about 60–80% circulating monocytes. It has been suggested that GCA possibly consists of two components: inflammatory reaction of the vascular wall and systemic monocyte activation, while in the case of PMR there probably is systemic monocyte activation without vasculitis (5).

Inflammation in the portal and lobular region of the liver with focal liver cell necrosis can be observed, sometimes accompanied with the formation of small epitheloid cell granulomas. Subtle inflammatory changes may be visible in the synovial tissue: the synovial fluid shows a slight inflammatory activity.

5

References

1.   Uddhammar A, Sundqvist KG, Ellis B et al. Cytokines and adhesion molecules in patients with polymyalgia rheumatica. Br J Rheumatol 1998; 37: 766–769.
2.   Balin H, Abdelmouttaleb I, Belmin J et al. Arterial wall production of cytokines in giant cell arteritis: results of a pilot study using human temporal artery cultures. J Gerontol A Biol Sci Med Sci 2002; 57: 241–245.
3.   Goronzy JJ, Weyand CM. Cytokines in giant-cell arteritis. Cleve Clin J Med 2002; 69: 91–94.
4.   Emilie D, Liozon E, Crevon MC et al. Production of interleukin 6 by granulomas of giant cell arteritis. Hum Immunol 1994; 39: 17–24.
5.   Wagner AD, Goronzy JJ, Weyand CM. Functional profile of tissue-infiltrating and circulating CD68+ cells in giant cell arteritis. Evidence for two components of the disease. J Clin Invest 1994; 94: 1134–1140.

Genetic factors in Giant Cell Arteritis and Polymyalgia Rheumatica

6

Vladimír Bošák

The etiopathogenesis of giant cell arteritis (GCA) and polymyalgia rheumatica (PMR) remains unknown, although genetic, autoimmune and environmental factors have been implicated. Evidence points to a genetic predisposition in these syndromes. GCA and PMR are more frequent in Caucasians, especially in the countries of northern Europe and in some regions of the United States, in those with Scandinavian ancestry (1, 2). Several cases of familial aggregation GCA and PMR have been also reported (3, 4) and HLA typing studies have shown a consistent association of both syndromes with certain alleles of the HLA system (5).

Attention to HLA antigens in GCA and PMR has been paid since 1975, when the first study was published (6). More than 40 various papers can be found in the literature focusing on this problem (5). HLA-A, B, C antigens have shown variable results, which suggests that a significant relationship is unlikely (5, 7, 8). Negative results were obtained also with respect to HLA-DQ (genes DQB1*, DQA1*) and HLA-DP antigens (5, 9). Positive findings were reported concerning HLA-DR antigens. GCA is the best example of an association between vasculitis and gene HLA-DRB1. Most studies have shown an association with alleles HLA-DRB1*04. PMR is associated with HLA class II genes, but this varies from population to another. Relapses of PMR, however, have been found to be significantly more common in patients who have the HLA-DRB1*04 alleles (5, 7, 8, 10, 11). The association between GCA/PMR and HLA-DR4 is typical predominantly for white Caucasian populations of Europe and North America, while such association could not be confirmed for Mediterranean populations – Italy, France (12, 13). Both PMR and antigen HLA-DR4 are rare in black populations. For Caucasians, frequencies of HLA-DR4 (HLA-DRB1*04) in the patients range between 36 and 71%, depending on the studied population. Most studies have described an association of PMR/GCA with alleles DRB1*0404/04 and DRB1*0401 (14, 10). Literature data also indicate an interaction between HLA-DRB1 and IL-4 that contributes to pronounced diseases susceptibility (15).

Attention was also paid to the relationships with clinical symptoms and laboratory findings in GCA and PMR. A majority of the studies brought negative results but some authors observed an association between HLA-DR4 antigen and visuals symptoms in GCA and GCA resistance to corticosteroid therapy. Thus, it cannot be ruled out that HLA-DR4 may be a marker of the severity of the disease (16).

It should be mentioned in connection with HLA-DR4 that this antigen is also associated with rheumatoid arthritis (RA), in particular with the prognostically more severe forms of the disease. RA setting on at older age ($\geq$ 60 years) on the other hand is clinically related to PMR, and it even seems to also have a similar immunogenetic characteristic – association with antigens HLA-DR1 and HLA-DR13/14 (9). Literary data suggest that PMR, GCA and RA may differ in their immunogenetic backgrounds (17). A lack of homozygosity or the shared epitope in GCA has been reported. This contrasts with observations in RA, in which homozygosity of the shared epitope is associated with more severe disease. The particular genetic locus in PMR/GCA has been mapped to the second hypervariable region (HVR2) of the HLA-DRB1 molecule (sequence motif spanning the amino acide positions 28-31 – DRYF). This HVR2 encodes sequences in the antigen-binding site of the floor of the HLA-DR molecule. However, this initial observation has not been confirmed in other populations from Europe (12, 13, 17).

Results of the study in the Slovak population confirmed a dominant role of HLA-DR4 (DRB1*04) in the predisposition to RA and GCA (18). A significantly increased frequency of the HLA-DR4 antigen was found in GCA (58%) compared with controls (21%, P < 0.01). The highest frequency of HLA-DR4 was observed in GCA patients with PMR (75%). HLA-DR4 was not associated with ESR, platelets count, alkaline phosphatase and visual symptoms in GCA. The relationship with DR4 was stronger in GCA (the relative risk RR = 5) than in RA (RR = 3). A more frequent occurrence of the HLA-DR4 antigen was observed in PMR (42%) but this difference was not significant (P > 0.05). The association with the HLA-DR1 antigen typical for Slovak RA patients (5) was not found in GCA and PMR. RA, GCA and probably also PMR are associated with the antigen HLA-DR4 in the Slovak population. Different alleles DRB1*04 or epitopes of the molecule HLA-DR4 probably participate on the predisposition to RA and PMR/GCA.

References

1. Baldursson O, Steinsson K, Bjornsson J, Lie JT. Giant cell arteritis in Iceland. An epidemiologic and histopathologic analysis. Arthritis Rheum 1994; 37: 1007–1012.
2. Salvarani C, Macchioni P, Zizzi F et al. Epidemiologic and immunogenetic aspects of polymyalgia rheumatica and giant cell arteritis in Northern Italy. Arthritis Rheum 1991; 34: 351–356.
3. Bartolome MJ, Martínez-Taboda VM, Lopez-Hoyos M et al. Familial aggregation of polymyalgia rheumatica and giant cell arterirtis. Clin Exp Rheumatol 2001; 19: 259–264.
4. Fietta P, Manganelli P, Zanetti A, Neri TM. Familial giant cell arteritis and polymyalgia rheumatica. Aggregation in 2 families. J Rheumatol 2002; 29: 1551–1555.
5. Bošák V. HLA-systém a jeho význam v reumatológii. In: Klinická reumatológia. 1. slov. vyd., Osveta, Martin 2000; 127–144 (in Slovak).
6. Rosenthal M, Mullen W, Albert ED et al. HL-A antigens in 15 patients with polymyalgia rheumatica and in 1142 controls. N Eng J Med 1975; 292: 595.
7. Gonzalez-Guy MA. Genetic epidemioliogy of GCA and PMR. Arthritis Res 2001; 3: 1554–1557.
8. Weyand MC, Goronzy JJ. Molecular approaches toward pathologic mechanism in GCA and Takayasu´s arteritis. Curr Opin Rheumatol 1995; 7: 30–36.
9. Gonzalez-Guy MA, Hajeer AH, Dababneh A et al. Seronegative rheumatoid arthritis in eldery and PMR have similar patterns of HLA association. J Rheumatol 2001; 28: 122–125.
10. Martínez-Taboda VM, Bartolome J, Lopez-Hoyos M et al. HLA-DRB1 allele distribution in polymyalgia rheumatica and giant cell arterirtis: Influence on clinical subgroups and prognosis. Semin Arthritis Rheun 2004; 34: 454–464.
11. Pease CT, Haugeberg G, Morgan AW et al. Diagnostic late onset rheumatoid arthritis, polymyalgia rheumatica and temporal arteritis in patients presenting polymyalgic symptoms. J Rheumatol 2005; 32: 1043–1046.
12. Reviron D, Foutrier C, Gula S et al. DRB1 alleles in PMR and rheumatoid arthritis in southern France. Eur J Immunogenet 2001; 28: 83–87.
13. Salvarani C, Boiardi L, Mantovani V, et al. HLA-DRB1 alleles associated with PMR in northern Italy: correlation with disease severity. Ann Rheum Dis 1999; 58: 303–308.
14. Gonzáles-Gay MA, Amoli MM, Garcia-Porrua C et al. Genetic markers of diseases susceptibility and severity in giant cell arteritis and polymyalgia rheumatica. Semin Arthritis Rheum 2003; 33: 38–48.
15. Amoli MM, Gonzales-Gay MA, Zeggini E et al. Epistatic interaction between HLA-DRB1 and interleukin 4, but not interferon-gama, increased susceptibility to giant cell arteritis. J Rheumatol 2004; 31: 2413–2417.
16. Gonzalez-Guy MA, Garcia-Porrua C, Hajeer AH et al. HLA-DRB1*04 may be a marker of severity in GCA. Ann Rheum Dis 2000; 59: 574–575.
17. Dababneh A, Gonzale-Gay MA, Garcia-Porrua C et al. GCA and PMR can be differentiated by distinct patterns of HLA class II association. J Rheumatol 1998; 25: 2140–2145.
18. Bošák V, Tuchyňová A, Rovenský J, Mičeková D. Immunogenetic study in Slovak patients with polymyalgia rheumatica and giant cell arteritis. Wien Med Wochenschr 2002; 152 (Suppl. 112): 9.

Polymyalgia rheumatica (PMR) and vascular complications

7

Viera Štvrtinová, Svetoslav Štvrtina, Jozef Rovenský

PMR is a syndrome closely associated with giant cell arteritis (GCA), and it is often considered a single disease (27). GCA can be found in about 50% of patients with PMR, and about 50% of PMR patients have positive findings in a temporal artery biopsy. Symptoms of PMR include morning stiffness, proximal muscle pain especially in the neck, shoulders and in the pelvis. The muscle pain is symmetric; muscles are pressure-sensitive without edema (37). The main complaint of PMR patients are morning stiffness with inability to stand up from the supine to the upright position, and inability to brush the hair. In cases of vasculitis affecting temporal artery and its branches, the pain is usually provoked by hairbrush contact with the inflamed artery wall.

GCA is a systemic granulomatous vasculitis of unknown etiology, typically affecting branches of carotid artery mainly temporal artery; however, any other medium or large artery can be affected. This fact complicates diagnosis of the disease.

Temporal arteritis is the most common form of GCA. In the 10th century, Ali Ibn Isa, an Arab ophthalmologist, recommended temporal artery excision in patients with migraines, who also had chronic eye disease progressing to vision loss (1). Clinically, Hutchins described temporal arteritis for the first time in 1890. Histopathological findings were correlated with the clinical syndrome by Horton in 1932. Only in 1938, Jenning recognized the loss of vision a disease complication (21). A few years later pathologist Gilmour found that temporal arteritis can affect any other arteries and named the disease "giant cell arteritis". GCA is a chronic inflammatory disease affecting medium a large arteries. Two main symptoms are present in the disease; temporal arteritis and PMR. William Bruce was the first who described PMR in 1888 (27). Nowadays, it is clear that GCA is a systemic disease with several serious, life-threatening cardiovascular complications. A diverse clinical presentation and a course of the disease are due to heterogeneous immune and inflammatory reactions (47). GCA most often affects branches of carotid artery, however, granulomatous panarteri-

7

tis can be found in any other medium or large-size artery. A term "temporal" is often used in quotes since it describes probable but not inevitable inflammation of temporal artery in GCA. The temporal artery can be affected in other diseases such as Wegener's granulomatosis or microscopic polyarteritis. On the other hand, the temporal artery is not necessarily affected in all patients with GCA (13). Temporal arteritis i.e. arteritis affecting temporal artery is not a deadly disease; patients life expectancy is comparable to the general population. GCA of large arteries can be, however, a lethal disease presented by a dissection or rupture of aorta in elderly (20, 41), as well as by a myocardial infarction or stroke (23). Unlike Takayasu arteritis, GCA is often found in 50+ years old patients, most often in 70 and 80 years olds. Recently, a juvenile form of the disease was confirmed by histological investigation (34, 36).

7.1
Incidence

In Göteborg, Sweden, an incidence of histologically-confimed GCA was found to be 5.5 per 100 000 or 16.8 cases of 50+ subjects (2). In Minnesota, USA, an average incidence of the disease increased from 5.1 per 100 000 in 1950s to 17.4 per 100 000 in the early 1970s (11). The increased incidence of GCA can be due to improved diagnostic of the disease. The GCA incidence of 2.2 per 10 000 was found in the Great Britain in 1990s. PMR incidence was found to be even higher; 8.4 per 10 000 (40); both disease often occurred in summer and were more frequent in southern parts of the country.

GCA is a disease often found in white Caucasians; it is relatively rare in other ethnic groups. The disease is two times more frequent in women than in men. The inflammation associated with the disease is more severe in women than in men and treatment time is longer in females (38). The majority of data on GCA and PMR are from studies in the Northern Europe and the North America.

7.2
Aetiology

The aetiology of the disease is unknown, however, a genetic predisposition and auto-immune mechanisms are often considered in the disease pathogenesis. Predominant occurrence in white Caucasians, family history, and an association with HLA-DR4 antigen is supportive of its genetic etiology (1, 18).

Immune cell mechanisms and deposition of immune complexes play an important role in the GCA pathogenesis. Increased concentrations of IgG, IgA and IgM were found in subjects with temporal arteritis. Antibody and complement deposits were confirmed by immunofluorescence in the affected arteries. Macrophages, epithelial-like cells and giant cells in arterial lesions produce various adhesion molecules such as ICAM-1. These findings suggest the inflammatory reaction in GCA depends on T cells reacting with antigens presented by tissue macrophages (8). Increased production of IL-1 beta and IFN-gamma appears to be an important factor modulating hyperplasia of intima in the affected blood vessels. Systemic concentrations of IL-6 are increased in GCA; whereas glucocorticoid therapy decreases IL-6 levels. Activation of blood mononuclear cells represents an additional mechanism to arteritis itself (12). Hypothyroidism with the presence of thyroid-specific antibodies was found in 10% of subjects with GCA (8).

The sudden onset of the disease and geographical differences in GCA and PMR incidence suggests that environmental factors play an important role in the disease pathogenesis. Olsson and coworkers (32) found an increased prevalence of GCA and PMR during two epidemics caused by *Mycoplasma pneumoniae*. The seasonal occurrence of PMR and GCA has been associated with epidemics of *chlamydia pneumoniae* and parvovirus B19 (33). Other possible mechanisms include seasonal changes of immune function causing variations in susceptibility to some diseases (38). Neuroendocrine mechanisms associated with aging can play a role in genetically predisposed individuals. Analysis of these changes is complicated by complex feedback relationships between inflammation and the neuroendocrine system. Good therapeutic response of glucocorticoids supports relative decrease in cortisol in PMR and GCA patients.

7.3
Histopathology

One of the typical findings in GCA is a granuloma i.e. focal inflammation in media of affected blood vessels, as seen in the case of 86 years old man (hematoxylin-eosin staining, Fig. 7). An inflammatory infiltration of histiocytes and plasma cells, less of lymphocytes and one giant multinuclear cell can be seen at higher magnification (Fig. 7). Elastic fiber structures disappear in the granuloma.

All vascular layers, in particular media, are affected in GCA. Splitting and fragmentation of the inner elastic membrane is typical for GCA (Fig. 9). Calcium deposition can be seen on the same picture in the area of the lamina elastica interna (Fig. 9). Another typical histologic finding for GCA is multinuclear giant cell (Figs. 8, 17, 20).

Focal inflammation consisting of giant cells affects blood vessel walls showing signs of smooth muscle atrophy and calcification in media. Typical deposits of calcium salts can be seen in lamina elastica interna of aorta in a biopsy from 84 years old woman (KOSSA staining, Fig. 15). Calcium deposition in lamina elastica interna is a typical finding in GCA.

Giant cells destroy inner elastic membrane and incorporate calcified parts of the membrane. Apparently, calcified parts of lamina elastica interna and an atrophy of media lead to inflammatory reactions (29). Calcifications of the inner elastic membrane are morphologically different from those in Monckeberg medial sclerosis, as well as from those in atherosclerosis, which are located in intima (31) (Fig. 14). Perhaps, these morphological differences cause accumulation of giant cells around calcifications in lamina elastica interna. An analysis of vascular segments not affected by inflammatory reaction showed more severe smooth muscle atrophy and calcifications of lamina elastica interna in GCA compared to healthy persons. The arteritis can be a result of metabolic changes in arterial wall, which leads to atrophy of smooth muscles in media, and to degeneration and calcification dystrophy of inner elastic membrane (30).

Giant cells present antigens for T cells, which subsequently produce cytokines. These cytokines attract macrophages, responsible for tissue damage in the affected artery by a production of reactive oxygen and nitrogen species and matrix metalloproteinases. The fragmentation of lamina elastica interna facilitates migration of fibroblasts causing hyperplasion, narrowing of vessel lumen and intense angiogenesis (48). Unlike normal arteries, in which vasa vasorum are limited to adventitia, in case of GCA, capillaries growth into media and intima (15).

Inflammatory damage in GCA is segmental. The intensity of inflammation varies in different parts of the same artery as well as between different blood vessels at different stages of the disease over time. Moreover, classic picture of granulomatous inflammation can be seen only in about 50% of patients; panarteritis with mixed inflammatory infiltrate consisting of polymorphonuclear leukocytes with some neutrophils or eosinophils without giant cells can be found in other patients (22). The panarteritis consists of leukocytes, lymphocytes and plasma cells, as depicted on Fig. 13 in case of our patient (hematoxylin-eosin staining).

7.4
Clinical picture of GCA

An onset and course of GCA is individual. Patients can suffer from headache or rheumatic joint and muscle difficulties similar to those of PMR (Table 4).

Typical features of disease are headache as well as painful swelling above temporal artery in elderly people (Fig. 1). As other medium or large arteries can be affected, clinical picture can vary accordingly. Other symptoms include nausea, lethargy, fever, claudication aching in jaws or tongue, chronic throat pain and painful scalp induration. Headache is usually localized in the area of temporal artery and it can radiate down into a neck, cheeks, jaw or tongue. Pressure sensitivity, induration, flushing and hair loss above temporal artery can develop later. An appearance of the first symptoms is usually acute, sometimes dramatic; however, some patients experience only general symptoms like weight loss, fever, weakness and anorexia. In the latter patients, the diagnosis can be very difficult.

Table 4   Clinical picture of the giant cell "temporal" arteritis

1.	Headache
2.	Painful induration and flush above temporal artery
3.	Claudication pain in jaw muscles and/or tongue
4.	Chronic throat pain
5.	Visual symptoms with following blindness
6.	Polymyalgia rheumatica
7.	Raynaud's phenomenon, paresthesias, claudication in extremities
8.	Dissecting aneurysm of aorta, rupture of aorta
9.	Signs of myocardial ischemia
10.	Signs of cerebral ischemia

The most serious complication of GCA is a vision loss occurring acutely and both eyes can be affected consecutively in a short-term interval (20). Although visual symptoms can appear rapidly resulting in a dramatic vision loss, the most of patients suffer for a few months from the permanent ophthalmologic symptoms such as vision impairment or blurred vision. This fact only accentuates a need for symptom search and immediate therapy. The vision loss is a consequence of ischemic neuritis of the optic nerve or the central retinal artery occlusion.

Damage of aorta and its branches is observed in approximately 10–15% patients with GCA and the symptoms of damage of large arteries include Raynaud's phenomenon, paresthesias and claudication in extremities. Life-threatening aorta damage can be a consequence of dissecting aneurysm of aorta or rupture of aorta (21). The macroscopic view of aorta curve area shows dissecting wall of aorta, in which blood sludge can be seen (Fig. 16). In the Fig. 12 displaying dissection in media, the blue color presents fibrin, which is an evidence for blood flow in false lumen of dissecting artery (phosphowolfram hematoxylin dye – 41). In patients with GCA the occurrence probability of thoracic aorta aneurysm is 17.3-fold higher and abdominal aorta aneurysm is 2.4 times higher (4).

Lesions of coronary arteries are not often presented, but in the literature there are data about deaths in consequence of acute myocardial infarction (16, 20, 26, 39). Damage of carotid and vertebrobasilar arteries can be manifested by cerebral infarction (1) as well as by other neurological symptoms such a distraction, dementia, depression, tinnitus, hearing impairment, mononeuritis multiplex, peripheral neuropathy and impairment of cranial nerves, e.g. paresis of oculomotor nerve (35).

Impairment of upper and lower extremities is rarely found in GCA. In upper extremities subclavic and brachial artery as well as their arterial branches are usually affected, in the lower extremities superficial femoral artery and popliteal artery are mainly affected. Clinically, it is manifested by appearance of claudications, eventually by sudden reduction in claudication distance. The claudication is mostly bilateral. Critical extremity ischemia is rarely found. In the literature only a small number of patients with extremity ischemia together with histologically confirmed findings of GCA is described so far (5, 6, 19, 44).

Life of patients is not significantly reduced by the presence of GCA provided that the disease is early and properly treated. Säve-Söderbergh (39) described the following causes of deaths in 9 patients with GCA – two patients died from myocardial infarction, two from dissecting aneurysm and five from a stroke. None of the described patients had adequate corticoid therapy.

7.5
Diagnosis

The principal symptoms of CGA include swollen and painful temporal artery, claudications in jaw muscles, blindness and PMR associated with high erythrocyte sedimentation rate. In laboratory testing, a higher erythrocyte sedimentation rate is observed in GCA (usually value of more than 50 mm/hour when using Westergren's method) as well as elevated C-reactive protein, normocytic normochromic anemia, elevated alkaline phosphatase, mildly elevated hepatic transaminases, elevated platelets and lower serum albumin (10). A few patients were described with low erythrocyte sedimentation rate (8). This is important in cases, when other symptoms indicate CGA diagnosis, hence a normal sedimentation rate does not delay the therapy.

In 1990 American College of Rheumatology developed classification criteria for CGA diagnosis (Table 5) based on a comparison of 214 GCA patients with a group of 593 patients with other forms of vasculitis (10). At least three of five classification criteria are necessary for diagnosis of GCA. The presence of three out of five criteria is associated with 93.5% sensitivity and 91.2% specificity for GCA diagnosis. An evaluation of the diagnostic criteria is simple, as, except of a biopsy, it requires only clinical examination. A biopsy is the only invasive method, performed in local anesthesia and it is associated with minimal complications.

Table 5   Classification criteria for CGA diagnosis
(According to American College of Rheumatology, 1990)

1.   Onset of disease in people older than 50 years
2.   Acute occurrence of localized headache
3.   Pressure painfulness of temporal artery or lower pulsation of temporal artery
4.   Higher erythrocyte sedimentation rate (over 50 mm/hour)
5.   Positive histological findings in biopsy

It is important to look for pathological changes in arteries, since the damage to large arteries can result in fatal consequences. It is also necessary to measure a blood pressure on both upper extremities. Ultrasound and angiographic examination are the methods enabling quantification of a artery system damage proportion (17). Typical ultrasound sign of GCA is mainly hypoechogenic ringlet ("halo") depicted around constricted lumen of the affected artery. Angiography shows smoothly outlined stenosis and mildly dilated segments, sometimes occlusions. While angiography identifies mainly changes of the artery lumen, the changes of the wall of large arteries are very well demonstrated by CT (9), MRI (25) and PET (44).

Final diagnosis is determined by a negative muscle biopsy and by findings of typical panarteritis in the biopsy of temporal artery, or an artery affected by other disease. Typical histopathological changes in GCA are a granulomatous inflammation, a presence of giant cells mainly in media, atrophy of smooth muscles and a destruction of elastic fibers, dissection and fragmentation of lamina elastica interna, as well as calcium deposition in lamina elastica interna and a new blood vessel growth (neovascularisation). As artery damage is segmental and biopsy does not have to hit an affected area, it is recommended to investigate more sections from 5–8 cm long segment of temporal artery (14), at least 2–3 cm long segment. If selected artery segment is negative in terms of presence of arteritis, but there is still clinical suspicion of GCA, it is necessary to examine temporal artery on the other side (22). The biopsy is important not only for confirmation of GCA diagnosis, but also for evaluation of disease activity. The biopsy should be performed before the corticosteroid treatment as it reduces the value of the examination. When the biopsy is done before the beginning of therapy, it can be useful in about 80% of cases; when the biopsy is performed in the first week of treatment, it is usually positive in about 60% of cases, however, when it is performed the week after the full glucocorticoid therapy, it is positive only in 20% of patients (27).

In differential diagnosis of patients without any histological confirmation of GCA diagnosis, it is essential to exclude malignant and infectious diseases, hypothyroidism and rheumatoid arthritis, as those diseases may be manifested by similar clinical or laboratory symptoms such PMR or GCA. In case of damage of large and medium arteries, it is necessary to consider possible contribution of atherosclerosis. It is important to note that arteries can be affected at the same time by vasculitis, as well as by atherosclerotic process (43).

7.6
Therapy

GCA is a very sensitive to glucocorticoid therapy. Withdrawal of muscle pain and rigidity in 24–48 hours after corticoid administration is actually a diagnostic test (28). Treatment should begin with the dose of 40 to 60 mg of prednisone with following consistent dose reduction of the drug to daily maintaining dosage of 7.5 to 10 mg, while it is necessary to increase the dose, when the symptoms reappear. A reduction of glucocorticoid dose should not be faster than 5 mg per week, and at the end of the first month it should not be lower than 20 mg per day. Sometimes it is necessary to use a higher dose than 60 mg in the form of pulse therapy, mainly in the case of vision impairment and threatening amaurosis (46).

Administration of glucocorticoids in a sufficient dose leads to withdrawal of clinical symptoms and to a decrease in erythrocyte sedimentation rate as the drugs improve the function of endothelial cells and reduce inflammatory response (7). GCA tends to have a fluctuating clinical course with alteration of periods of exacerbation and remission of the disease. Glucocorticoids are effective in suppression of clinical symptoms of GCA and also in prevention of visual impairment. However, already existing impairment of vision is irreversible (20). The glucocorticoid therapy is usually used in combination with vasodilatation and antithrombotic therapy. In patients suffering from PMR it is advantageous to add non-steroidal antireumatic drugs in the therapy.

As there is no laboratory test predicting therapy effectiveness, recommended average therapy duration varies among studies. Although in some patients glucocorticoids during the first 6 months can be sufficient, the recommended time of therapy is at least 2 years in total. As 20–50% of patients treated by glucocorticoids suffer from side effects e.g. compression vertebral fractures in 26% of patients, it is still necessary to find a drug dose sufficient enough but with minimal side effects (8). According some authors a milder or more "benign" form of GCA exists, when there is an administration of lower dosage of prednisone (45). After the initial dose of 40 mg of prednisolone daily, Bengtsson (1) gradually reduced the dose to 2.5 mg daily and this was followed by a withdrawal of prednisone treatment when after a month of such a minimal maintaining dosage clinical symptoms did not reappear. However, a relapse occurs in about 50% of patients on such a therapy regime and it is necessary to restart prednisone therapy again in a dose of 10–15 mg daily with gradual reduction to 2.5–5 mg daily during one or two months.

A combined therapy of glucocorticoids with azathioprine is used rarely with possibility to lower glucocorticoids doses. According some case observations in patients resistant to glucocorticoids, methotrexate was proved effective in GCA therapy as well. In some cases of extracranial GCA, it is possible to use also interventional radiological or surgery methods, e.g. angioplasty in the therapy (3).

GCA significantly increases a risk of aorta aneurysm presenting often as a late fatal complication of the disease. Therefore, it is necessary to actively search for aneurysm in all patients; to perform regularly duplex ultrasound examination, CT or MRI scans. It is also necessary to adhere very strictly to the treatment regime. The majority of cases with a preceding history of GCA were on low doses of steroid or on no treatment at the time of dissection and the median erythrocyte sedimentation rate of these patients was 62 mm per hr (24). It is also important to treat hypertension since high blood pressure was found in almost 77% of patients with dissecting aorta. Untreated or insufficiently treated hypertension is one of the important factors contributing to occurrence of dissecting aortic aneurysm.

References

1. Bengtsson, B.A.: Giant cell arteritis. In: The vasculitides. Science and practice. (Eds.: B.M. Ansell, P. A. Bacon, J.T. Lie, H. Yazici), Chapman and Hall Medical, London – Glasgow – Weinheim – New York – Tokyo – Melbourne – Madras 1996, 171–180.
2. Bengtsson, B.A., Malmvall, B.E.: The epidemiology of giant cell arteritis including temporal arteritis and polymyalgia rheumatica. Arthritis Rheum., 24, 1981, 899–904.
3. Both, M., Aries, P.M., Muller-Hulsbeck, S. et al: Balloon angioplasty of upper extremity in patients with extracranial giant cell arteritis. Ann. Rheum. Dis., 65, 2006, 9, 1124–1130.
4. Evans, J.M., O´Fallon, W.M., Hunder, G.G.: Increased incidence of aortic aneurysm and dissection in giant cell (temporal) arteritis. A population – based study. Ann. Intern. Med., 122, 1995, 7, 502–507.
5. Dupuy, R., Mercié, P., Neau, D. et al: Giant cell arteritis involving the lower limbs. Rev. Rheum., 64, 1997, 500–503.
6. Garcia Vázques, J.M., Carreira, J.M., Seoane, C. et al.: Superior and inferior limb ischemia in giant cell arteritis: angiography follow up. Clin. Rheumatol., 18, 1999, 61–65.
7. Gonzales-Juanatey, C., Llorca, J., Garcia-Porrua, C. et al.: Steroid therapy improves endothelial function in patients with biopsy. proven giant cell arteritis. J. Rheumatol., 33, 2006, 1, 74–78.
8. Hellmann, D.B.: Immunopathogenesis, diagnosis, and treatment of giant cell arteritis, temporal arteritis, polymyalgia rheumatica, and Takayasu's arteritis. Curr. Opin. Rheumat., 5, 1993, 25–32.
9. Herve, F., Choussy, V., Janvresse, A. et al.: Aortic involvement in giant cell arteritis. A prospective follow-up of 11 patients using computed tomography. Rev. Med. Interne, 27, 2006, 3, 196–202.
10. Hunder, G.G., Bloch, D.A., Michel, B.A. et al.: The American College of Rheumatology 1990 criteria for the classification of the giant cell arteritis. Arthritis Rheum., 33, 1990, č. 8, 1122–1128.
11. Huston, K.A., Hunder, G.G., Lie, J.T. et al.: Temporal arteritis. A 25 year epidemiologic, clinical and pathologic study. Ann. Intern. Med., 88, 1978, č. 2, 162–167.
12. Imrich, R., Bošák, V., Rovenský, J.: Polymyalgia rheumatic a temporálna arteritída: vzťah hormónov k patogenéze. Rheumatologia, 17, 2003, č.1, 69–77.
13. Jennette, J.Ch., Falk, R.J., Andrassy, K. et al.: Nomenclature of systemic vasculitides. Proposal of an International Consensus Conference. Arthritis. Rheum., 17, 1994, č. 2, 187–192.
14. Joyce, J.W.: Arteritis. In: Arterial Surgery. (Ed: H.H.G. Eastcott), Churchill Livingstone, Madrid – Melbourne – New York – Tokyo 1992, 211–222.
15. Kaiser, M., Younge B., Bjornsson, J., et al.: Formation of new vasa vasorum in vasculitis. Production of angiogenic cytokines by multinucleated giant cells. Am. J. Pathol., 155 (3), 1999, 765–74.
16. Karger, B., Fechner, G.: Sudden death due to giant cell coronary arteritis. Int. J. Legal Med., 120, 2006, 6, 377–379.
17. Kolossváry, E., Kollár, A., Pintér, H. et al.: Bilateral axillobrachial and external carotid artery manifestation of giant cell arteritis: important role of color duplex ultrasonography in the diagnosis. Int. Angiol., 24, 2005, 2, 202–205.
18. Lee, S.J., Kavanaugh, A.: Autoimmunity, vasculitis and autoantibodies. J. Allergy Clin Immunol., 117, 2006, 2, S445–S450.
19. Le Hello, C., Lévesque, H., Jeanton, M. et al.: Lower limb giant cell arteritis and temporal arteritis: follow up of 8 cases. J. Rheumatol., 28, 2001, 6, 1407–1411.
20. Lie, J.T., Failoni, D.D., Davis, D.C.: Temporal arteritis with giant cell aortitis, coronary arteritis, and myocardial infarction. Arch. Pathol. Lab. Med., 110, 1986, č. 9, 857–860.
21. Lie, J.T.: Coronary vasculitis. A review in the current scheme of classification of vasculitis. Arch. Pathol. Lab. Med., 111, 1987, 3, 224–233.
22. Lie, J.T.: Illustrated histopathologic classification criteria for selected vasculitis syndromes. Arthr. Rheum., 33, 1990, č. 8, 1074–1087.

7

23. Lie, J.T.: Aortic and extracranial large vessel giant cel arteritis: a review of 72 cases with histopathologic documentation. Semin. Arthritis Rheum., 24 (6), 1995, 422–31.

24. Liu, G., Shupak, R., Chiu, B.K.: Aortic dissection in giant cell arteritis. Semin. Arthritis Rheum., 25, 1995, 3, 160–171.

25. Markl, M., Uhl, M., Wieben, O. et al.: High resolution 3T MRI for the assessment of cervical and superficial cranial arteries in giant cell arteritis. J. Magn. Reson. Imaging, 24, 2006, 2, 423–427.

26. Martin, J.F., Kittas, C., Triger, D.R.: Giant cell arteritis of coronary arteries causing myocardial infarction. Br. Heart. J., 43, 1980, č. 4, 487–489.

27. Murphy, E.A., Capell, H.: Aortitis and large vessel vasculitides. In: A Textbook of Vascular Medicine. (Eds: J.E. Tooke, G.D.O. Lowe), Arnold, London – Sydney – Auckland, 1996, 287–294.

28. Nesher, G., Sonnenblick, M.: Steroid-sparing medications in temporal arteritis – report of three cases and review of 174 reported patients. Clin. Rheumat. 13, 1994, č. 2, 289–292.

29. Nordborg, C., Nordborg, E., Petursdottir, V.: The pathogenesis of giant cell arteritis: morphological aspects. Clin. Exp. Rheumatol., 18, (4 Suppl. 20), 2000 a, S18–21.

30. Nordborg, C., Nordborg, E., Petursdottir, V.: Giant cell arteritis. Epidemiology, etiology and pathogenesis. APMIS, 108 (11), 2000 b, 713–24.

31. Nordborg, C., Nordborg, E., Petursdottir, V. Fyhr, I.M.: Calcification of the internal elastic membrane in temporal arteries:its relation to age and gender. Clin. Exp. Rheumatol., 19 (5), 2001, 565–568.

32. Olsson, A., Elling, P., Elling, H.: Synchronous variations of the incidence of arteritis temporalis and polymyalgia rheumatic in different regions of Denmark; association with epidemics of Mycoplasma Pneumoniae infection. Clin. Rheumat., 13, 1994, č. 2, 384.

33. Perfetto, F., Moggi-Pignone, M., Becucci et al.: Seasonal pattern in the onset of polymyalgia rheumatica. Ann. Rheum. Dis., 64, 2005, 1662–1663.

34. Pipinos, I.I., Hopp, R., Edwards, W.D., Radio, S.J.: Giant cell temporal arteritis in a 17-year-old male. J. Vasc. Surg., 43, 2006, 5, 1053–1055.

35. Polak, P., Pokorny, V., Stvrtina, S. et al.: Temporal arteritis presenting with paresis of the oculomotor nerve and polymyalgia rheumatica, despite a low erythrocyte sedimentation rate. J. Clin. Rheumatol., 11, 2005, 4, 242–244.

36. Rovenský, J., Tauchmannová, H., Štvrtinová, V., Štvrtina, S.: Príspevok k problematike juvenilnej temporálnej arteritídy. Rheumatologia, 19, 2005, 4, 153–155.

37. Rovenský, J., Tauchmannová, H., Štvrtinová, V., Štvrtina, S., Duda J.: Polymyalgia rheumatica a obrovskobunková arteritída, príspevok ku klinicko-laboratórnej syndromológii a terapii. Čes. Revmatol., 14, 2006, 3, 135–143.

38. Rovenský, J., Štvrtinová, V., Tauchmannová, H., Duda, J.: Polymyalgia rheumatica and giant cell arteritis – importance of factors contributing to severity of disease. Rheuma 21st, Archived Reports – www.rheuma21st.com/archives/cutting

39. Säve-Söderbergh, J., Malmvall, B.E., Andersson, R., Bengtsson, B.A.: Giant cell arteritis as a cause of death. JAMA, 255, 1986, č. 4, 493–496.

40. Smeeth, L., Cook, C., Hall, A.J.: Incidence of diagnosed polymyalgia rheumatica and temporal arteritis in the United Kingdom, 1990 to 2001. Ann. Rheum. Dis., 65, 2006, 8, 1093–1098.

41. Štvrtina, S., Rovenský, J., Galbavý, Š.: Aneuryzma aorty ako príčina smrti pri obrovskobunkovej arteritíde. Rheumatologia, 17, 2003, 3, 213–220.

42. Štvrtinová, V.: Primárne systémové vaskulitídy. SAP 1998, Bratislava, 210.

43. Štvrtinová, V., Rauová, Ľ., Tuchyňová, A., Rovenský, J.: Vasculitis of the coronary arteries and atherosclerosis: random coincidence or causative relationship? In: Atherosclerosis and Autoimmunity. (Eds: Y. Shoenfeld, D. Harats, G. Wick), Elsevier, Amsterdam – Lausanne – New York – Oxford – Shannon – Singapore – Tokyo 2001, 315–327.

44. Tato, F., Hoffmann, U.: Clinical presentation and vascular imaging in giant cell arteritis of the femoropopliteal and tibioperoneal arteries. Analysis of four cases. J. Vasc. Surg., 44, 2006, 1, 176–182.

45. Ter Borg, E.J., Haanen, H.C., Seldenrijk, C.A.: Relationship between histological subtypes and clinical characteristics at presentation and outcome in biopsy proven temporal arteritis: Identification of a relatively benign subgroup. Clin. Rheumatol., 2006, Jul 1.

46. Tuchyňová, A., Rovenský, J., Mičeková, D.: Polymyalgia rheumatica a temporálna arteritída – klinický obraz a liečba. Rheumatologia, 12, 1998, 3, 117–122.

47. Weyand, C.M., Goronzy, J.J.: Pathogenetic principles in giant cell arteritis. Int. J. Cardiol., 75, 2000, Suppl. 1, S9–S15.

48. Weyand, C.M., Goronzy, J.J.: Pathogenetic mechanisms in giant cell arteritis. Cleve. Clin. J. Med., 69, Suppl. 2, 2002, SII28–32.

Chronobiology of Polymyalgia Rheumatica and Giant Cell Arteritis

8

Howard Bird

8.1
Introduction

Chronobiology, which is the study of biological rhythms, is perhaps unduly neglected within medicine. It assumes particular importance for diseases, many of them rheumatic diseases and polymyalgia rheumatica [PMR] in particular, where there is clear evidence of a diurnal variation in symptoms. The dramatic improvement in early morning stiffness such that it is invariably abolished by lunchtime even figures in diagnostic criteria sets for PMR.

Current thinking suggests that the diurnal variation in endogenous cortisol has evolved for the more efficient functioning of the human body during daylight hours and that this is probably mediated through other neuronal and hormonal pathways, with melatonin [MLT] a prime candidate. Such pathways are closely linked with diurnal variation in cytokines, which probably largely accounts for diurnal symptomology in rheumatic diseases since, as a group, these inflammatory conditions are cytokine-driven.

In addition to influencing symptoms, diurnal rhythms have important implications for dosing, not just of non-steroidal anti-inflammatory drugs [NSAIDs] but particularly for the dosing of steroids, which at present remains the backbone of treatment in this condition.

The literature also contains reference to a seasonal variation in the incidence of PMR, though this is harder to study because of confounding factors such as the seasonal availability of health care in certain developed countries.

8

8.2
Other Rheumatic Conditions

Circadian rhythms have long been recognised in rheumatoid arthritis [RA] (1). In this condition, pain and stiffness become clinically more apparent overnight such that they are maximum at about 0500 hours, reducing gradually thereafter during the next day. This has implications both for function (e.g. grip strength) and in discomfort and disability (2). Circadian rhythms have also been identified in other rheumatic diseases, including polymyositis, which is associated with a circadian variation in serum myoglobin levels (3).

The way in which this links with hormones has been discussed for some 20 years (4, 5). An intricate association between neuro-endocrine effect, sex hormones and symptoms is accepted. In the last decade, interest has additionally centred not only on cortisol but also cytokines, particularly interleukin-6 [IL-6], which many consider to be one of the principal cytokines mediating PMR and giant cell arteritis [GCA] (6).

8.3
Mechanisms of Variation

Here, the evidence, drawn largely from RA but possibly to some extent applicable to PMR, becomes a little confusing. It is no surprise that in RA circadian variation in grip strength differs in phase by about 12 hours from circadian variation in inflammation, grip strength strongest towards the late afternoon. The circaseptan rhythm (about 7 days) of paw oedema observed in animal models (7) probably lacks relevance however.

Endogenous corticosteroids and MLT are both undoubtedly implicated. In adult primates visible light, observed by the subject, influences the hypothalamic region of the brain that directs circadian rhythms. Deprivation of observed light modifies the circadian rhythm for many neuro-hormones, particularly cortisol and MLT. In normal subjects, MLT peaks at about 0300 hours whereas cortisol peaks at 0400 hours. Interleukins tend also to peak overnight and then remain low throughout the day. There also seems to be a differential effect in interleukins, overnight variation in IL-6 and cortisol both more marked than variation in TNFα or other cytokines (6).

In RA an early surge in plasma ACTH correlates closely with increased IL-6 (8) and Th-1 type cytokine also increases significantly with a peak that is even slightly earlier (1).

MLT serum levels are significantly higher in patients with RA than in controls (9) and there is even a suggestion of variation in the diurnal rhythm across Europe. Thus, when IL-6 and TNFα concentrations were observed in RA in patients from Estonia and Italy at 0400 hours and midnight, Estonian patients displayed higher cytokine levels than Italian patients, implying latitude may have an influence though this is not necessarily the only explanation for the higher prevalence in RA in northern Europe than in Mediterranean countries. The higher prevalence of PMR in Scandinavia, sometimes alternatively attributed to either genetic clustering or local infection, comes to mind.

8.4
Diurnal Variation in Polymyalgia Rheumatica/Giant Cell Arteritis

The presence of severe early morning stiffness figures prominently in several diagnostic criteria sets (10, 11, 12) as well as in the recently proposed disease activity score for monitoring response to treatment (13).

Studies on cytokine and steroid levels in PMR have been justified largely because of diagnostic confusion between PMR and elderly onset RA [EORA]. In a study of PMR, EORA and a third group of patients felt to represent EORA with a specific PMR-like onset, TNFα, IL-6, IL-1 receptor antagonist levels as well as steroid levels, were compared together with levels in a group of control patients (14). Serum IL-6 was significantly higher in both PMR and EORA/PMR than in EORA or control, whereas IL-1 receptor antagonist serum levels were significantly higher in patients with EORA than in controls and levels highest in patients with PMR and EORA/PMR. After glucocorticoid treatment, serum TNFα and IL-6 levels significantly decreased in all patient groups. It was argued that patients with PMR and with EORA/PMR have a more intense inflammatory reaction and might be more efficient responders to glucocorticoid treatment than patients with EORA, though a group of patients with classical RA alone was not included in this study.

It remains uncertain whether the seasonal pattern in the onset of PMR reflects a function of chronobiology or has an alternative explanation. In a study from Italy (15), a winter peak of incidence was once again identified, perhaps suggesting an infective aetiology at that time of year.

8.5
Implications for Steroid Therapy

Against the above biological background, there has been recent intense interest in the most rational method of delivering glucocorticosteroid therapy. A workshop under the auspices of the EULAR Standing Committee on International Clinical Studies had first addressed this as early as 2002 (16). This considered not only pharmacological variation between the different steroid analogues available commercially (17) (though in practice prednisolone is invariably used by the oral route of administration) but also considered timing of dosing in relation to the circadian rhythm of endogenous cortisol production and in the diurnal variation of symptoms. It considered frequency of dosing during the day, though did not specifically consider PMR. It also accepted that answers derived from consensus conferences were not definitive. It was noted, however, that in view of the relative hypocorticolism that occurs in PMR, glucocorticoid treatment might be as much replacement therapy for reduced adrenal production as supplementary therapy (18). Although this work was largely directed at RA it may still have implications for PMR.

Consideration should also be given to the precise formulation of the administrated steroid and its reliability of release. There is a strong anecdotal impression that release from enteric-coated formulations of prednisolone is unreliable and erratic compared to a non-enteric formulations. Some patients not responding to enteric-coated prednisolone respond immediately when non-enteric coated prednisolone is substituted at the same dose. Against this background, there is evidence that in RA low doses of prednisolone taken at 0200 hours have more effect on severe morning symptoms than when the same dose is taken at 0730 hours, which might be expected, although the required awakening in the middle of the night may itself influence diurnal control. Alternative slow release preparations, seemingly reliable, if taken at bedtime in RA release the drug automatically around 0200 hours with corresponding improvement on morning stiffness (19). Use of this formulation in PMR has been recommended (20), but not yet studied.

Treatment with alternate-day steroids has been proposed to reduce the risk of adverse reactions but has been associated with a higher dose of treatment phase (21).

Although NSAIDs are felt by the majority not to have a place in the management of PMR, it has been known for many years that a 4-fold improvement in tolerance and a doubling of analgesic effectiveness can accrue as a result of varying the ingestion time of indomethacin (22).

References

1. Cutolo M, Seriolo B, Craviotto C, Pizzorni C, Sulli A. Circadian rhythms in RA. Ann Rheum Dis 2003; 62: 593–596.
2. Bellamy N, Sothern RB, Campbell J, Buchanan WW. Circadian rhythm in pain, stiffness, and manual dexterity in rheumatoid arthritis: relation between discomfort and disability. Ann Rheum Dis 1991; 50: 243–248.
3. Bombardieri S, Clerico A, Riente L, Del Chicca MG, Vitali C. Circadian variations of serum myoglobin levels in normal subjects and patients with polymyositis. Arthritis Rheum 1982; 25: 1419–1424.
4. Bhalla AK. Hormones and the immune response. Ann Rheum Dis 1989; 48: 1–6.
5. Kirkham BW, Panayi GS. Diurnal periodicity of cortisol secretion, immune reactivity and disease activity in rheumatoid arthritis: implications for steroid treatment. Rheumatol 1989; 28: 154–157.

6.   Perry MG, Kirwan JR, Jessop DS, Hunt LP. Overnight variations in cortisol, interleukin 6, tumour necrosis factor α and other cytokines in people with rheumatoid arthritis. Ann Rheum Dis 2009; 68: 63–68.

7.   Loubaris N, Cros G, Serrano JJ, Boucard M. Circadian and circannual variation of the carregeenin inflammatory effect in the rat. Life Sci 1983; 32: 1349–1354.

8.   Crofford LJ, Kalogeras KTRL. Circadian relationships between interleukin(IL)-6 and ypothalamic-pituitary-adrenal axis hormones: Failure of IL-6 to cause sustained hypercortisolism in patients with early untreated rheumatoid arthritis. J Clin Endocrinol Metab 1997; 82: 1279–1283.

9.   Cutolo M, Maestroni GJM. The melatonin-cytokine connection in rheumatoid arthritis. Ann Rheum Dis 2005; 64: 1109–1111.

10.   Bird HA, Esselinckx W, Dixon AS, Mowat AG, Wood PH. An evaluation of criteria for polymyalgia rheumatica. Ann Rheum Dis 1979; 38: 434–439.

11.   Chuang T-Y, Hunder GG, Ilstrup DM, Kurland LT. Polymyalgia Rheumatica: A 10-Year Epidemiologic and Clinical Study. Ann Intern Med 1982; 97: 672–680.

12.   Healey LA. Long-term follow-up of polymyalgia rheumatica: Evidence for synovitis. Semin Arthritis Rheum 1984; 13: 322–328.

13.   Leeb BF, Rintelen B, Sautner J, Fassl C, Bird HA. The polymyalgia rheumatica activity score in daily use: Proposal for a definition of remission. Arthritis Care Res 2007; 57: 810–815.

14.   Cutolo M, Montecucco CM, Cavagna L, Caporali R, Capellino S, Montagna P, Fazzuoli L. Villaggio B, Seriolo B, Sulli A. Serum cytokines and steroidal hormones in polymyalgia rheumatica and elderly-onset rheumatoid arthritis. Ann Rheum Dis 2006; 65: 1438–1443.

15.   Perfetto F, Moggi-Pignone A, Becucci A, Cantini F, Di Natale M, Livi R, Tempestini A, Matucci-Cerinic M. Seasonal pattern in the onset of polymyalgia rheumatica. Ann Rheum Dis 2005; 64: 1662–1663.

16.   Buttgereit F, Da Silva JAP, Boers M, Burmester G-R, Cutolo M, Jacobs J, Kirwan J, Köhler L, van Reil P, Vischer T, Bijlsma JWJ. Standardised nomenclature for glucocorticoid dosages and glucocorticoid treatment regimens: Current questions and tentative answers in rheumatology. Ann Rheum Dis 2002; 61: 718–722.

17.   Straub RH, Cutolo M. Review: Involvement of the hypothalamic-pituitary-adrenal/gonadal axis and the peripheral nervous system in rheumatoid arthritis: Viewpoint based on a systemic pathogenetic role. Arthritis Rheum 2001; 44: 493–507.

18.   Arvidson NG, Gudbjörnsson B, Larsson A, Hällgren R. The timing of glucocorticoid administration in rheumatoid arthritis. Ann Rheum Dis 1997; 56: 27–31.

19.   Buttgereit F, Doering G, Schaeffler A, Witte S, Sierakowski S, Gromnica-Ihle E, Jeka S, Krueger K, Szechinski J, Alten R. Efficacy of modified-release versus standard prednisolone to reduce duration of morning stiffness of the joints in rheumatoid arthritis (CAPRA-1): A double-blind randomised controlled trial. Lancet 2008; 371: 205–214.

20.   Bijlsma JWJ, Jacobs JWG. Glucocorticoid chronotherapy in rheumatoid arthritis. Lancet 2008; 371: 183–184.

21.   Hunder GG, Sheps SG, Allen GL, Joyce JW. Daily and alternate-day corticosteroid regimens in treatment of giant cell arteritis: Comparison in a prospective study. Ann Intern Med 1975; 82: 613–618.

22.   Reinberg A, Lévi F. Clinical chronopharmacology with special reference to NSAIDs. Scand J Rheumatol 1987; 16 (Supp. 65): 118–122.

Histopathology of Giant Cell (temporal) Arteritis – changes in aorta

9

Svetoslav Štvrtina, Jozef Rovenský

9.1
Introduction

Giant cell arteritis (GCA) is a systemic granulomatous vasculitis of unknown etiology, that, typically, involves the branches of carotid artery (especially of temporal artery), but it can involve any medium-size or large artery, and then its diagnosis becomes much more difficult (1). Temporal arteritis is the most frequent form of giant cell arteritis. It is characteristic by affecting the branches of carotid artery ("temporal" artery). The name "temporal" is quoted in inverted brackets because it expresses frequent, but not always involvement of temporal artery in this disease. The temporal artery can also be affected with the disease process in other forms of vasculitis, e.g. Wegener granulomatosis or microscopic polyarteritis. On the contrary, inflammation of temporal artery is not necessarily manifested in all the patients with giant cell arteritis (2).

Temporal arteritis (i.e. arteritis involving temporal artery) is not a lethal disease; the patients live the same average age as a normal population. However, giant cell arteritis, that involves medium-size and large arteries, can be lethal and it is often manifested in a dramatic way, via dissection or rupture of aorta in the elderly, but also by myocardial infarction or emergency cerebral accident (3). From clinical point of view, temporal arteritis was described for the first time in 1890 by Hutchinson. The histopathological picture related to clinical syndrome was outlined in 1932 by Horton (Fig. 5), but it was as late as 1938, when Jenning recognised that, blindness can be a grave complication of the disease (4). Later Gilmour, a pathologist, showed that, temporal arteritis can involve also other arteries and he was the first to use the term "giant cell arteritis" (GCA). In the clinical picture, two different sets of symp-

9

toms can be recognised – the first being temporal arteritis and the second polymyalgia rheumatica, described for the first time by William Bruce in 1888 (5). Today it is
clear that GCA is a systemic condition with many severe, life-threatening cardiovascular complications. Its manifold and varying clinical picture and course of the
disease is probably caused by the heterogenity of both immune and inflammatory
reaction in specific patients (6).

The aim of our work is to discuss typical histopathologic changes in the aorta of
GCA patients.

9.2
Case reports

Case 1

An 86-year old patient with history of coronary artery disease and peptic ulcer,
after anteroseptal *myocardium* infarction two years ago was admitted to the hospital for chest pain lasting for two hours. At the time of the admission his blood
pressure was 90/60 mm Hg, and the ECG showed a picture of acute myocardial
infarction of the anterior wall. Urgent thrombolysis could not be carried out in
the patient because of melaena, probably due to bleeding from a duodenal ulcer.
18 hours after admission to the hospital, the patient suddenly died.

The autopsy revealed a fresh extensive myocardial infarction of the anterior
and posterior wall of the left ventricle and of papillary muscles of mitral valve.
When examining the abdominal aorta, two circular (ring-like) widenings of lumen (aneurysms) were observed below the renal artery branches, and both the
iliac arteries were extended in a balloon-like way having 1.2 cm in the diameter
(Fig. 6). One of typical histopathologic findings in GCA is a granuloma, or
granulomatous inflammation of the media, as we can see in the figure 7 in the
abdominal aorta in our 86-year old man (stained by hematoxyline – eosine –
HE). The inflammatory infiltrate contained mostly histiocytes and plasmatic
cells, but few lymphocytes and one giant multinucleated cell can be seen
(Fig. 7). In the area of granuloma the structure of elastic fibres disappears. The
typical multinucleated giant cell is on the figure 8. All the layers of the vessel
wall are involved, but the media the most. The inner elastic membrane was spit
and fragmented, as it is visible in the figure 9 in the same patient. Figure 9
shows also a calcium deposition in the area of lamina elastica interna. In other
histologic picture from aorta of the same patient (Fig. 10) we can see typical
multinucleated giant cells.

Case 2

An 84-year old woman with the history of arterial hypertension and coronary artery disease, admitted to a hospital for quantitative disturbance of consciousness (sopor to coma) with 110/70 mm Hg blood pressure. ECG showed sinus bradycardia (with 50/min frequency) with no signs of an acute coronary accident. Her blood count showed severe anaemia (haemoglobin – 5.4 g/l) and leucocytosis (11×10^9/l). Cerebral CT did not show any fresh ischaemic or haemorrhagic lesion. The patient died after 6 hours of hospitalisation.

Macroscopic examination during her autopsy discovered a 3.5 cm long longitudinal tear at the posterior wall of aorta 2 cm above the aortal valve. The tear made a haematoma cavity between adventitia and media. The cavity continued to abdominal aorta, and there, at the level of truncus coeliacus, a crosswise 1 cm long fissure was found at the posterior wall of aorta through which the blood poured back to the lumen of aorta. A dissecting aneurysma of ascending thoracic aorta, that continued to the descending thoracic and abdominal aorta (Fig. 11) was the cause of death of the patient. The histological investigation of the aortic wall revealed that aneurysm developed due to giant cell arteritis. A dissection in media, where blue color represents fibrin, a proof of blood flowing in the false lumen of the dissecting aneurysm, can be seen in the Fig. 12 (phosphowolfram haematoxyline staining). Panarteritis with mixed inflammatory infiltrate (Fig. 13) was found in some parts of the aorta, whereas the other parts show atrophy of smooth muscles of media together with pronounced calcifications. Typical deposits of calcium salts in aorta of our patient (Fig. 14) can be seen in the area of lamina elastica interna (KOSSA staining); in the intima we can see atherosclerotic plaque with calcium. Figure 15 shows calcium deposition in the area of lamina elastica interna in the same patient.

Case 3

An 81-year old patient with the history of two myocardial infarctions with an implanted pacemaker was admitted to hospital for strong, intense pressure pain across a large area in the front part of chest. ECG showed a pacemaker rhythm with frequency of 70/min, and the condition after anteroseptal and lateral myocardial infarction. His values of indicating enzymes of myocardium damage – CK, AST, ALT – were normal, just as his blood count. After twenty hours of hospitalisation suddenly both his breathing and heart stopped and the clinician supposed another acute heart attack.

9

At autopsy, a four cm long longitudinal tear was discovered at the superior wall of aorta, 0.4 cm above the aortal valve. The tear made a sac between the adventitia and media 8 cm long, filled with dark red clots (Fig. 16). The cause of death in this patient was giant cell arteritis with dissecting aneurysm of ascending aorta. The fresh myocardial infarction supposed by clinician was not proven by autopsy. The histological pictures of this 86 year old patient's aorta showed mixed inflammatory infiltrate (Fig. 17) and neovascularisation (Fig. 18) in the media of aorta with inflammatory infiltration and destruction of elastic fibres of media.

9.3
Discussion

Involvement of aorta and its branches is found in about 10-15% GCA patients. This involvement can be life-threatening due to development of dissecting aneurysm or rupture of aorta (4). GCA is one of the most common vasculitis in population over the age of 50 years. Evans et al (7) found that patients with GCA were 17.3 times more likely to develop a thoracic aortic aneurysm and 2.4 more likely to develop an abdominal aortic aneurysm compared with the general population. In a population-based study of a cohort of patients with GCA aortic aneurysm and/or dissection developed in 18% (30 incident cases from 168 patients in the cohort) (8). In some patients a concomitant giant cell aortitis, aortic aneurysm and aortic arch syndrome could be present (9).

The character of inflammatory damage in GCA is segmental. The intensity of inflammatory response differs in different parts of the same vessel and in individual vessels, and it varies in different stages of the disease as well (10). The classical picture of granulomatous inflammation with giant cells is observed in 50% patients; the other half of patients with positive histological finding show panarteritis with mixed inflammatory infiltrate that is mainly of lymphomononuclear character with some neutrophils and eosinophils, but with no giant cells (11). Such panarteritis, developed into mixed inflammation consisting of polymorphonuclear leucocytes, lymphocytes and plasmocytes is clear from the Fig. 13. Two stages of inflammation are discerned in GCA (12) In atrophic arterial segments a focal, foreign-body, giant-cell reaction to the calcified internal elastic membrane was found, but in other biopsies a different picture with a diffuse macrophage attack on media and intima with numerous and apparently macrophage-derived giant cells, which did not attack calcification was seen. Morphologically, the inflammatory process appears to be initiated by a foreign-body giant cell attack on calcified internal elastic membrane in arteries and on calcified atrophic parts of the aortic media. The ensuing diffuse chronic inflammation leads to vessel wall dilatation and extensive intimal thickening. The latter, which relates to the production of promoting factors by the inflammatory cells, causes arterial stenosis and ischemic complications 13).

Giant cells obviously "attack" inner elastic membrane and incorporate the calcified parts of the membrane. It seems that calcification in the area of the lamina elastica interna and the atrophy of media are inevitable prerequisites for development of inflammatory response (14). Calcification of the inner elastic membrane differs morphologically from the calcification developed in Monckeberg mediosclerosis, and from atherosclerotic calcifications (15). This is shown also in the Fig. 14 and this morphological difference will probably be a reason that giant cells start gather around calcium in lamina elastica interna. The analysis of vessel segments that are not affected by the inflammatory response showed a significantly greater atrophy of smooth muscles of media, and also calcifications in the area of inner elastic membrane compared with the group of healthy volunteers. The involvement of arteries at the beginning of disease can be caused by metabolic disorders in the arterial wall. That gradually leads to the atrophy of smooth muscles of media, and to degeneration and dystrophic calcifications of the inner elastic membrane. Giant cells developing around foreign corpuscles come probably from smooth muscles and then they respond to the presence of degenerated and calcified inner elastic membrane (13). Because of the high age of patients with GCA, vasculitis can set in the vascular wall already damaged by the atherosclerotic process and the inflammatory response can be triggered by so far unknown mechanism (16). Thus in patients with GCA we can see together atherosclerotic as well as vasculitic changes as it is evident from Fig. 14 and 15, where incorporation of calcium to lamina elastica interna is a typical sign of vasculitis and atherosclerotic plaque in the intima layer is characteristic sign of atherosclerosis.

T cells emerge as the key players in inflammation-associated injury pathways. In GCA, all injury mechanisms have been related to effector macrophages. Macrophages in the adventitia focus on production of proinflammatory cytokines. Macrophages in the media specialize in oxidative damage with lipid peroxidation attacking smooth muscle cells and matrix component. These macrophages also supply reactive oxygen intermediates that, in combination with nitrogen intermediates, cause protein nitration of endothelial cells. Production of oxygen radicals is complemented by production of metalloproteinases, likely essential in the breakdown of elastic membranes. With the fragmentation of lamina elastica interna, the intimal layer becomes accessible to migratory myofibroblasts that later cause hyperplasia of intima and occlusion of the vessel lumen (17). Development of hyperplastic intima is accompanied by intensive neoangiogenesis. While in normal arteries the presence of vasa vasorum is restricted to adventitia, in the case of inflamed arteria the capillaries grow into media and intima (18). Neoangiogenesis is present also in the aorta of our 86-year-old patient (Fig. 18).

The diagnosis of GCA is made through characteristic histological finding, revealed at biopsy of temporal artery; or from the material taken during surgery (19). Because involvement of the vessels is segmental, meaning that biopsy may not happen to hit the right spot, bioptical examination of several cuts is recommended: the sections shall be taken from 5–8 cm big area temporal artery (20), the minimum being 2–3 cm big spot. If the selected area of artery gives a negative result in biopsy, i.e. no arteritis can be proven, but there is still clinical suspicion of GCA, examination of temporal artery on the other side is recommended (11). Biopsy should be carried out before the therapy is started, since corticoid treatment decreases the value of bioptic examination (11). If biopsy is done before the therapy starts, it is beneficial in 80% of cases; if it is made in the first week of treatment, it is still positive in 60% of cases; however, a biopsy carried out a week after full treatment by corticoids, it is positive only in 20% of patients (5).

The survival of patients is not significantly shortened by the presence of giant cell arteritis (21), under the condition that the disease is early enough and properly treated. Säve-Söderbergh et al. (10) describe following causes of death in 9 GCA patients – two patients died of myocardial infarction, two of dissecting aneurysm and five of sudden cerebral accident. None of the patients described was administered adequate corticoid therapy. Lie (3) reports 18 patients with extracranial GCA, with these causes of death: rupture of aortal aneurysm in 6 patients, dissection of aorta in 6 patients, cerebral infarction in 3 patients and myocardial infarction in 3 patients.

Because involvement of large arteries in GCA can have fatal consequences, in all patients it is recommended to look for changes in these arteries in a focused way. Blood pressure shall be measured in both upper extremities. Methods that enable to judge the extent of arterial system affliction include ultrasound and angiographic examination. GCA significantly increases the risk of development of aortal aneurysm that often presents a late complication of a disease that may cause death of patients. That is why it is necessary to actively seek aneurysms in all GCA patients – make regular duplex ultrasonography examinations, CT or MR examinations if possible, too. Patients with diagnosed GCA shall be carefully and properly treated, since in most of the patients in which aortal dissection developed the treatment was not adequate.

9.4
Conclusion

Giant cell arteritis involving aorta, can be a lethal disease and it is often manifested in a dramatic way in the elderly: by dissection or rupture of aorta. Early diagnostics, correct treatment and life-long checks of patients in whom GCA was diagnosed can prevent them from development of such a severe complication as aortic aneurysm.

Typical histopathologic changes in GCA include granulomatous inflammation, presence of giant cells – especially in media, atrophy of smooth muscles and destruction of elastic fibres, splitting and fragmentation of lamina elastica interna, as well as deposition of calcium salts into the area of lamina elastica interna, diffuse inflammation of vessel wall and ingrowth of capillaries (neovascularisation).

References

1. Štvrtinová V. Primary Systemic Vasculitides. Slovak Academic Press, Bratislava 1998; 210 pp (in Slovak).
2. Jennette JCh, Falk RJ, Andrassy K et al. Nomenclature of systemic vasculitides. Proposal of an International Consensus Conference. Arthr Rheum 1994; 17: 187–192.
3. Lie JT. Aortic and extracranial large vessel giant cel arteritis: a review of 72 cases with histopathologic documentation. Semin Arthritis Rheum 1995; 24 (6): 422–431.
4. Lie JT. Coronary vasculitis. A review in the current scheme of classification of vasculitis. Arch Pathol Lab Med 1987; 111 (3): 224–233.
5. Murphy EA, Capell H. Aortitis and large vessel vasculitides. In: A Textbook of Vascular Medicine (eds. Tooke JE, Lowe GDO), Arnold, London – Sydney – Auckland 1996; 287–294.
6. Weyand CM, Goronzy JJ. Pathogenetic principles in giant cell arteritis. Int J Cardiol 2000; 75 (Suppl1): S9–S15.
7. Evans JM, O'Fallon WM, Hunder GG. Increased incidence of aortic aneurysm and dissection in giant cell (temporal) arteritis: a population based study. Ann Intern Med 1995; 122: 502–507.
8. Nuenninghoff DM, Hunder GG, Christianson TJH et al. Incidence and predictors of a large-artery complication (aortic aneurysm, aortic dissection, and/or large-artery stenosis) in patients with giant cell arteritis. Arthritis Rheumat 2003; 48: 3522–3531.
9. Nuenninghoff DM, Warrington KJ, Matteson EL. Concomitant giant cell aortitis, thoracic aortic aneurysm, an aortic arch syndrome: Occurrence in a patient and significance. Arthritis Rheumat (Arthritis Care and Research) 200; 49: 858–861.
10. Säve-Söderbergh J, Malmwall BE, Andersson R, Bengtsson BA. Giant cell arteritis as a cause of death. JAMA 1986; 255 (4): 493–496.
11. Lie JT. Illustrated histopathologic classification criteria for selected vasculitis syndromes. Arthritis Rheum 1990; 33 (8): 1074–1087.
12. Nordborg E, Bengtsson BA, Nordborg C. Temporal artery morphology and morphometry in giant cell arteritis. APMIS 99, 1991; 1013–1023.
13. Nordborg C, Nordborg E, Petursdottir V. Giant cell arteritis. Epidemiology, etiology and pathogenesis. APMIS 2000; 108 (11): 713–724.
14. Nordborg C, Nordborg E, Petursdottir V. The pathogenesis of giant cell arteritis: morphological aspects. Clin Exp Rheumatol 2000; 18 (4 Suppl 20): S18–21.
15. Nordborg C, Nordborg E, Petursdottir V, Fyhr IM. Calcification of the internal elastic membrane in temporal arteries: its relation to age and gender. Clin Exp Rheumatol 2001; 19 (5): 565–568.
16. Štvrtinová V, Rauová Ľ, Tuchyňová A, Rovenský J. Vasculitis of the coronary arteries and atherosclerosis: Random coincidence or a causative relationship? In: Atherosclerosis and Autoimmunity (eds. Shoenfeld Y, Harats D, Wick G), Elsevier, Amsterdam – Lausanne – New York – Oxford – Shannon – Singapore – Tokyo 2001; 315–327.
17. Weyand CM, Goronzy JJ. Pathogenetic mechanisms in giant cell arteritis. Cleve Clin J Med 2002; 69 (Suppl 2): SII28–32.
18. Kaiser M, Younge B, Bjornsson J et al. Formation of new vasa vasorum in vasculitis. production of angiogenic cytokines by multinucleated giant cells. Am J Pathol 1999; 155 (3): 765–774.
19. Bengtsson BA. Giant cell arteritis. In: The Vasculitides. Science and Practice (eds. Ansell BM, Bacon PA, Lie JT, Yazici H), Chapman and Hall Medical, London – Glasgow – Weinheim – New York – Tokyo – Melbourne – Madras 1996; 171–180.
20. Joyce JW. Arteritis. In: Arterial Surgery (ed. Eastcott HHG), Churchill Livingstone, Madrid – Melbourne – New York – Tokyo 1992; 211–222.
21. Huston KA, Hunder GG, Lie JT et al. Temporal arteritis. A 25 year epidemiologic, clinical and pathologic study. Ann Intern Med 1978; 88: 162–167.

Ultrasonography in Polymyalgia Rheumatica and/or Giant Cell Arteritis

10

Peter Poprac, Jozef Rovenský

The recent technical advances in ultrasonography (US) allowed the use of the method for a differential diagnosis of many diseases and to distinguish between normal and abnormal tissues. The color duplex US with Doppler system enable us to gain information not only on pathological changes in joints, but also to evaluate changes of the blood vessels in patients with PMR and GCA. A small effusion or synovium thickening in the affected joints and an amount of vascularization in synovium, both signs of inflammation, can be analyzed using the US imaging.

US is a relatively simple and rapid imaging technique for effusion detection in the joints. An ultrasonographic distance between the hip joint capsule of 7 mm and more, or a difference between the hips of 1 mm or more, are regarded positive for hip joint effusion. An intraarticular effusion is present in the glenohumeral joint when the distance between joint capsule and the head of the humerus is more than 3.5 mm, or the difference between both sides is 1 mm or more. An effusion in the knee joint is positive when the suprapatelar recessus is dilated more than 2 mm. Koski (1) found pathological changes in the glenohumeral joints by US in 19 patients with PMR, and in 12 of them the effusion was detected as well. Frediani (2) observed shoulder effusion in the subacromial-subdeltoidal bursae, tendosynovitis of the long head of biceps tendon and in glenohumeral joint in about 70% patients with PMR.

GCA is a common inflammatory vasculopathy of large and medium-size arteries, especially those branching from the proximal aorta. In 1990, the American College of Rheumatology developed classification criteria for GCA (3). Schmidt and colleagues recently proposed that the color duplex US has a role in the diagnosis of temporal arteritis (TA) (4). The authors of the latter study showed an evidence for a dark halo around lumen of the temporal arteries. The finding, possibly be due to oedema of the artery wall, was the most specific sign of TA on US. The authors suggested that in the setting of typical signs of GCA, the clear halo allowed the diagnosis of the disease without performing temporal artery biopsy. However, the study did not compare US with physical examination of temporal arteries. It also did not clearly evaluate whether US may be useful in patients with PMR or systemic illness in the absence of definitive clinical signs of GCA (5).

The primary objectives are to assess the value of US in the diagnosis of GCA. Salvarani (6) found that ultrasonographic evidence of the dark halo around the lumen of the temporal arteries had a sensitivity of only 40%. The absence of the dark halo on US neither ruled out nor substantially decreased the likelihood of biopsy.

The US image of the inflamed temporal artery is characterized by:

> *Edema* – a dark hypoechoic (not anechoic) circumferential wall thickening "halo" appearing around the lumen of the temporal artery. The halo usually disappears after 2–3 weeks of corticosteroid treatment.
> *Stenosis* – a narrowing of vessel lumen leads to increased blood flow velocities and turbulence. The color Doppler US shows a mixture and a persisting color signaling in the diastole. Doppler curves confirm this finding if the blood flow velocity is more than twice the rate recorded in the area before the stenosis and reduced velocity behind the area of stenosis.
> *Occlusion* – images delineates the temporal artery with absence of color signal in it. Pulsatility of inflamed artery is often reduced (6).

10.1
Patients and results

During the period of 2005–2006 a total of nineteen patients with PMR were examined using US (Acuson 128 XP/10c, with the 5–7,5 MHz linear probe) in the NURCH. All the patients underwent US of the glenohumeral, hip and knee joints.

An intraarticular effusion in the glenohumeral joint or in the biceps tendon sheath and in the subdeltoid bursa respectively (Fig. 19), was detected in 13 untreated patients (68%). The effusion was presented as a small residuum in six patients (35%) after 6 months therapy with corticosteroids. The intraarticular effusion in the hip (Fig. 20) was detected in 7 untreated patients (41%) and in 5 treated patients (29%). Small effusion was present in the knee joint of 7 untreated patients and in 7 patients (38%) treated with corticosteroids. Analysis of synovial fluid was made in 5 patients. Cells in synovial fluids were in range of 300–10 400.

The incidence of GCA in patients with PMR is highly controversial. In patients without clinical signs of GCA ("pure PMR") it ranges between 0%–41%. The most authors do not recommend temporal artery biopsy to be performed routinely in patients with "pure PMR". As an alternative examination the US with color mode can be performed. The US was done before biopsy in GCA patients by the author using a 7.5 MHz linear probe on the Acuson 128 XP/10c. The arteries were examined as extensively as possible in transverse and longitudinal sections and pulsatility, resistivity indices. In a group of 5 patients with GCA, the image of temporal artery wall edema was present in 2 patients in the acute stage of TA (Figs. 21, 22). The other patients were treated in the time of their US examination.

10.2
Discussion

GCA is a condition that involves inflammation of arteries, and is common in older patients of 60 years of age and more. Very often this condition is called temporal arteritis due to a frequent involvement of the temporal arteries. A severe complication of GCA is a loss of vision. Diagnosis of GCA can be difficult without a biopsy of the temporal artery. The biopsy is a minor surgical procedure that allows doctors to obtain a piece of tissue, which is subsequently examined under a light microscope. Some reports have suggested that ultrasound tests of the temporal artery can be helpful in diagnosing GCA, but the role of US in diagnosis of this condition remains uncertain. The US involves using sound waves to take special pictures (7). The authors analyzed studies published up to April 2004 in the MEDLINE, EMBASE and Cochrane databases, reference lists, and direct contact with investigators. The aim was to determine the diagnostic value of US for GCA diagnosis. A sensitivity as well as specificity of the halo sign, stenosis and occlusion were analyzed in 23 studies involving a total of 2036 patients, fulfilling the inclusion criteria. Limitations of the meta-analysis are the small number of patients in the primary studies, modest quality and considerable heterogeneity. Also our group of patients has been very small and heterogeneous in terms of therapy. In conclusion, our results suggest a presence for more than 1 mm around the vessels increased the likelihood of a diagnosis of GCA based on a biopsy test.

References

1.   Koski JM. Ultrasonographic evidence of synovitis in axial joints in patients with polymyalgia rheumatica. Br J Rheumatol 1992; 31: 201–203.
2.   Frediani B, Falsetti P, Storri L et al. Evidence for synovitis in active polymyalgia rheumatica: sonographic study in larges series of patients. J Rheumatol 2002; 29 (3): 644.
3.   Hunder GG, Bloch DA, Michel BA et al. The American College of Rheumatology 1990 criteria for the clasification of giant cell arteritis. Arthritis Rheum 1990; 33: 1122–1128.
4.   Schmidt WA, Kraft HE, Vorpahl K et al. Color duplex ultrasonography in the diagnosis of temporal arteritis. N Engl J Med 1997; 337: 1336–1342.
5.   Hunder GG, Weyand CM. Sonography in giant–cell arteries. N Engl J Med 1997; 337: 1385–1386.
6.   Salvarani C, Silingardi M, Ghirarduzzi A et al. Is duplex ultrasonography useful for the diagnosis of giant-cell arteritis. Ann Intern Med 2002; 137: 232–238.
7.   Karassa FB, Matsagas MI, Schmidt WA, Ioannidis JPA. Meta-analysis: Test performance of ultrasonography for giant-cell arteritis. Ann Int Med 2005; 142: 359–369.

Therapy of Polymyalgia Rheumatica and Giant Cell Arteritis

11

Jozef Rovenský, Richard Imrich

Polymyalgia rheumatica and giant cell arteritis (PMR a GCA) are undoubtedly diseases with exceptionally good response to glucocorticoid treatment. Significant improvement after the administration of glucocortioids can be seen within 48 hours after the treatment is started. However, it is necessary to observe all the principles required for glucocorticoid treatment. Glucocorticoid daily dose normally does not exceed 15 mg, but the potential of a lower initial dose has been also reported. On the other hand, some authors consider a 10 mg dose insufficient as they needed the dose of 15–20 mg to keep the disease in remission. The goal of treatment is to reach at least partial remission within the first 4 weeks of the disease. The effect of treatment is evaluated after the first month of treatment. The clinical prednisone dose is most often decreased by 2.5 mg every 4 weeks. Doses of 5 to 7.5 mg of prednisone should be used as maintaining doses and patients should receive them at least for 12 months. In some patients, it is necessary to continue usually for 2 years, or 4 to 5 years in some cases. It is necessary to note that the positive effect of glucocorticoids can be limited by their adverse effects. Daily doses not exceeding 5 mg are relatively safe. However, the situation is different with PMR as we expect the administration of glucocorticoids taking more than 6 months with doses exceeding 5 mg. Therefore, it is necessary to use the appropriate complex examination, including bone densitometry, and to observe the respective laboratory parameters to monitor the appearance of osteoporosis. Prophylactic calcium and vitamin-D therapy, as well as biphosphonate therapy in appropriate cases, is also important. Non-steroidal antirheumatic drugs are useful for treatment, but not as first-line drugs. They are administered with a low dose of glucocorticoids until the disease activity is managed. In GCA treatment, therapy is launched with high daily doses of prednisone (40 to 80 mg), mainly in patients with visual impairment and imminent blindness. Sometimes it is necessary to use a more intensive dose format – pulse therapy. Doses should not be decreased faster than 5 mg per week and at the end of the first month the dose should not be lower than 20 mg. Lower doses presumably

11

enable reactivation of basic disease and the increase of mortality among patients at the same time. Sometimes, combined therapy with azathioprine or leflunomide is also used for treatment that could enable application of lower corticosteroid doses. According to some case studies of patients resistant to glucocorticoid therapy, methotrexate worked well, however, we do not know for sure whether lower glucocorticoid doses can be used under this combination of drugs. However, GCA treatment must be long-term (at least 2 years) and glucocorticoid therapy also should be ceased not earlier than after 2 years of treatment.

Nowadays, anti-cytokine treatment is being considered on the basis of the pathogenesis of GCA. First reports focused their attention to infliximab and etanercept. Cantini et al. (2001) used them in 4 GCA patients with a severe form of the disease and a failure to reach remission with long-term glucocorticoid treatment. Reduction of the daily dose of glucocortioids to 7.5 to 12.5 mg a day resulted in the relapse of disease, and severe adverse effects such as osteoporosis, fractures, diabetes and phacoscleroma occurred in all 4 patients. In these 4 patients, the following infliximab dosage regimen has been used: infliximab was to be administered in 3 intravenously infused doses of 3 mg/kg in week 0, 2, 6 and the results proved that complete clinical and humoral remission was reached after 2 weeks of the described above treatment. In 3 patients clinical remission was maintained without any steroidal therapy after 6, 5 and 5 months from the infusion of the 3rd dose. The fourth patient did not responded sufficiently and the treatment was ceased after 2nd infusion. Despite of partial response after 1st infusion relapse in the form of increased sedimentation and CRP values occurred in the patient at the time of 2nd infusion. It cannot be excluded that the patient would have got better if the infliximab dose had been increased. The drug was well tolerated. In 2007, Salvarini et al. published a survey on the effect of infliximab combined with prednisone, or placebo with prednisone, for patients with newly occurred PMR. They pointed out that the administration of a small dose of infliximab with prednisone compared to the group of PMR patients treated with prednisone alone has not resulted in any differences in the occurrence of relapse of the disease between those two groups. Similar negative results in PMR treatment has also been reported by Hoffmann at al. (2005) in patients with newly occurred PMR with the similar study design (1st group placebo plus glucocorticoids, 2 group infliximab (5 mg/kg) plus glucocorticoids) using the same time intervals as in the previous study. After 22 weeks of treatment, these two groups differ neither in the occurrence of relapse nor in the dose of glucocorticoids. In 2007, Catanazo et al. reported the possibilities of etanercept therapy for the resistant form of PMR. They dealt with patients with relapsing form of PMR with no possibility to reduce the daily prednisone dose below 7.5 to 10 mg and with the occurrence of adverse effects of corticosteroids. Etanercept was applied to these patients for 24 weeks in the dose of 25 mg twice a week and they were monitored during the next 3 months after the therapy was ceased. In all 6 patients remission was maintained, in 4 patients the improvement reached 70% according to the EULAR criteria. In 2 patients the improvement reached 50%. Results were evaluated at the end of the 9 months long study. Also, the important reduction of a cumulative dose of prednisone was proved in the group receiving etanercept treatment compared to the control group. Authors indicated that etanercept could be a safe and useful drug for patients with relapsing PMR enabling the reduction of gluco-corticosteroids. Also, Ahmed et al. reported in 2007 on the possibility of adalimumab therapy for patients with resistant forms of GCA. The study dealt with an old woman aged 70 with a severe for of temporal arteritis treated with 60 mg daily dose of predni-sone. Despite of initial improvement (regression of headache) and stabilization of eye-related symptoms, 1 week later the condition of the patient got worse due to persistent headache, tiredness and deteriorated vision in left eye. Methylprednisolone was ad-ministered to the patient for 3 days in the daily dose of 1 g with the follow-up 20 mg dose of peroral prednisolone 3 times a day. Despite of clinical improvement reached at the daily dose of 40 mg with 12.5 mg of methotrexate, the patient was admitted to hospital due to serious deterioration of her condition (productive cough, pleuritic murmur and increased tiredness). Methotrexate therapy was immediately ceased, but simultaneously, vision in the left eye got worse and the CRP level increased, so that pulsion methylprednisolone therapy was launched with the daily dose of 1 g for 3 days and with the subsequent increase of the prednisone daily dose to 60 mg. Despite the improvement in the patient's condition, steroidal diabetes developed and in Septem-ber 2005 adalimumab therapy was started. 6 months after the adalimumab therapy was commenced the patient was asymptomatic and the prednisolone daily dose was decreased to 12.5 mg.

However, monoclonal antibody against IL-6 might also be used in future and there-fore studies searching for the ways how to block its production can be expected. Based on the findings with respect to suprarenal androgens substitution with dihydroepian-drosteron sulphate is also being considered for future. However, it is necessary to point out that current trends in medicine are evidence-based and therefore the ideas of anti-cytokine therapy in PMR and GCA, as well as of hormonal substitution mentioned above, have been only used to outline possible future developments of treatment.

Diagnostic Criteria, Treatment, and Monitoring of Polymyalgia Rheumatica/Giant Cell Arteritis

12

Burkhard F. Leeb, Thomas Nothnagl, Martin Steindl, Bernhard Rintelen

Usually, PMR shows an acute, in any case a rapid, onset with severe and symmetric, muscle pain in the shoulder girdle and the neck, less often in the pelvic girdle, accompanied by muscle tenderness. Patients suffer from continuous pain often aggravated during physical inactivity or the night. Sometimes transient synovitis occurs without radiological signs of arthritis. Polymyalgia rheumatica is frequently accompanied by a number of non-specific symptoms, such as lethargy, depression fatigue, and fever, loss of appetite and weight, and overall weakness. William Bruce was the first to describe the disease, naming it senile gout in 1888 (1) However, there is no specific positive finding that confirms the disease therefore a variety of criteria sets for the diagnosis of PMR GCA have been developed targeting reasonable sensitivity and specificity.

The first criteria set to be formally proposed was a multi-collaborative one from 11 United Kingdom rheumatology units in 1979, which led to the Bird/Wood criteria (2). This was soon followed by two further criteria sets (from Jones and Hazleman in 1981 (3) and from Chuang et al. in 1982 (4), both of which were more based on clinical expertise than on epidemiological analyses. In 1985 Wilke et al. (5) developed diagnostic criteria primarily targeted to diagnose GCA, whereas the Nobunaga criteria of 1989 (6) were designed specifically for a Japanese population and circumstances.

In 1997 a European collaborative PMR-working group was initiated by ESCISIT (EULAR Standing Committee on Clinical Trials including Therapeutic Trials). One of the two objectives of this task force was a sensitivity analysis of the existing diagnostic criteria sets, as mentioned above, by the means of a Pan-European observation. The other one was the development of PMR-response criteria in order to provide a possibility to monitor the disease process and the therapeutic success (7, 8).

The European collaborative PMR group comprised 8 centers covering all parts of the continent (Leeds, UK; Stockerau, AUT; Ljubljana, SLO; Kaunas, LIT; Pavia, ITA; Jerusalem, ISR; Tartu, EST; Piestany, SLK). 213 patients were enrolled into the diagnostic criteria validation study (7).

All patients were interviewed with respect to a full medical history and examined physically, evaluating all the features of existing diagnostic criteria (2–6). The diagnosis of PMR was finally established by experienced clinicians.. The Bird/Wood (2) criteria performed best with a sensitivity of 99.5%, with the Chuang-Hunder (3) criteria achieving the second place, with a sensitivity of 93.3%, in identifying patients from this group of 213 patients considered suffering from PMR by ten experienced investigators

Table 6   Bird/Wood Criteria (2)

1.   Bilateral Shoulder Pain and/or Stiffness
2.   Duration of Onset of 2 Weeks or Less
3.   Initial Esr >40 Mm/Hour
4.   Duration Early Morning Stiffness >one Hour
5.   Age 65 Yrs or More
6.   Depression and/or Weight Loss
7.   Bilateral Upper Arm Tenderness
Probable Pmr: any 3 or More of these Criteria   *or* <3 Criteria with a Clinical Abnormality of Temporal Artery
Further Proposed: Definite Pmr Would be Probable Pmr with a Positive Response to Steroid Therapy using a Single Blind Therapeutic Test of Steroid Against Placebo

Table 7   Chuang Hunder Criteria (4)

1.   Patient age >50 yrs
2.   Bilateral aching
3.   Tenderness for one month or more
i.   of neck or torso   ii.   shoulders or upper arms iii.   and hips or thighs
4.   ESR > 40 mm/hour 5.   Exclusion of other diagnosis
Definite PMR if a patient complies all of the criteria mentioned above

Table 8   1990, American College of Rheumatology (ACR) criteria for classifying GCA (9)

1.   age above 50,
2.   Newly occurred headache,
3.   Tenderness or decreased temporal artery pulsation,
4.   Increased erythrocyte sedimentation rate exceeding 50 mm/hour,
5.   Biopsy-proven necrotizing arteritis with mononuclear infiltrate or granulomatous infiltrate usually with multinuclear giant cells.
GCA can be classified if 3 of the 5 classification criteria are fulfilled at a sensibility of 93.5% and specificity of 91.2%.

from all across Europe (7). Of four criteria sets compared these both performed significantly better than the two other criteria sets, though each of these was admittedly developed for rather specialized reasons. The identification range was found to be between 99.5% (Bird-Wood) and 67.8% (Nobunaga) for the sets of criteria applied (7). Thus both criteria sets, providing more than 90% sensitivity during this observation, namely the Bird-Wood criteria, and the Chuang-Hunder criteria, can be recommended for diagnosing PMR in daily routine as well as in clinical trials.

In 1990, the American College of Rheumatology (ACR) published the following criteria for classifying GCA (9). The patient can be classified as suffering from GCA if 3 of the 5 classification criteria are fulfilled, achieving a sensibility of 93.5% and specificity of 91.2%.

12.1
Treatment

Polymyalgia rheumatica and giant cell arteritis are diseases with an exceptionally favorable response to glucocorticoid treatment. It is well known and overall consensus that corticosteroid therapy usually leads to a rapid and dramatic improvement of patients' complaints and returns them to previous functional status (10, 11). Almost immediate pain relief after initiation of corticosteroids can be regarded an additional diagnostic feature for PMR (2). If no significant pain reduction can be achieved by an adequate steroid dose, the diagnosis has to be seriously reconsidered.

However, neither corticosteroids nor alternative treatments have been studied in a controlled way up to now, with respect to initial dosing and duration of therapy (8). The dosages used initially vary to a high degree and are based rather on experience than on evidence. The recently published EULAR response criteria for PMR and the PMR-disease activity score were developed on the basis of corticosteroid treatment (8, 12). As expected patients showed a quick and impressive response after the initiation of corticosteroids during these studies. The initial dose amounted to a mean of 24.68 (+/– 28.61 SEM) mg prednisolone equivalent, indicating a high variability of the starting doses applied in the single centers. The initial dose could be tapered down to a mean of 7.68 (+/– 3.61 SEM) mg at week twenty-four (p < 0.0001). The corticosteroid response time was evaluated by asking the patient for the onset of improvement after the first corticosteroid dose and amounted to 35, 4 hrs +/– 18, 93 (8).

Nevertheless, it is mandatory to consider all risks for and contraindications of glucocorticoid treatment. The long term daily glucocorticoid doses applied for the purpose of PMR treatment does not usually exceed 15 mg. Lower initial doses have been also reported in a number of publications. However, some authors consider 10 mg/day as an insufficient dose insufficient, because maintaining the disease in remission was only possible administering 15 to 20 mg/day. The current experience considers an initial dose from 25 to 15 mg prednisone/day the most appropriate one. The therapeutic effect should be evaluated after one month of treatment as the goal of initial treatment is to achieve remission during the first 4 weeks of disorder. In daily practice, we reduce the corticosteroid dose 2.5 mg of prednisone every 4 weeks. Maintenance daily prednisone doses should not exceed 5 to 7.5 mg and should be applied for at least 12-month period. Some patients must be kept on treatment for 2 years and a little percentage even for 4 to 5 years. However, in these patients the diagnosis of PMR should be reevaluated cautiously, particularly with respect to eventually existing rheumatoid arthritis (13). During the course of treatment a step-by-step reduction of the daily corticosteroid dose is recommended in accordance to the clinical situation, and the acute phase response parameters, both combined by the Polymyalgia rheumatica activity score (PMR-AS) (12). It is also well known that relapses may occur frequently during the course of the disease despite ongoing corticosteroid therapy (10, 11). Cautious and slow tapering of the corticosteroid dosage may prevent those relapses; however, as with corticosteroid therapy for PMR in general, there is an urgent need for more evidence in this aspect (10).

The severity of PMR shows high variations. In corticosteroid-refractory cases and to avoid corticosteroid related side effects drugs such as methotrexate (MTX), and azathioprine (AZA), have been suggested as corticosteroid sparing agents, and have been investigated in a few clinical trials with sometimes inconclusive results (14, 15, 16). Both of them are reported to be beneficial in patients resistant to corticosteroid treatment. However it is not completely clarified yet to what extent glucocorticoid doses can be reduced by administering such combinations.

Recently, the application of tumor necrosis factor (TNF)-blockers in corticosteroid refractory patients or those experiencing side effects, such as hyperglycemia was considered. First investigations dealing with infliximab and etanercept treatment (17, 18) presented highly promising results, however, the initial results for infliximab could not be upheld in controlled studies (19), whilst a single controlled study with etanercept in GCA was positive but not indeed convincing due to the number of patients included (20). For adalimumab only a few case studies have been published. As a perspective for the future, the application of a monoclonal antibody against the interleukin-6 receptor, namely tocilizumab, could give beneficial therapeutically results, given some investigative findings (21).

In some less severe cases of PMR treatment with Nonsteroidal Antirheumatic Drugs (NSAIDs) may be sufficient to control the disease effectively (22, 23), Sometimes they are applied in combination with low-dose glucocorticoid treatment. However, recent knowledge about the risk of NSAIDs with respect to coronary artery disease and hypertension, and well established evidence concerning the risk for – in part life-threatening – gastrointestinal side effects, may lead to reconsideration of the long-term application of these drugs in the respective population (24).

GCA treatment should be started applying high daily prednisone doses of 40 to 80 mg, especially in patients with visual disturbances and impending amaurosis. Sometimes higher doses are deemed necessary in form of pulse treatment. Prednisone doses should not be reduced by more than 5 mg per week and the daily dose at the end of the first month should not be lower than 20 mg, otherwise GCA may often be reactivated with an increase of the mortality rate. One possibility to spare glucocorticoids may be given by simultaneous AZA or MTX treatment (25, 26, 27). Both of them are reported to be beneficial in patients resistant to corticosteroid treatment. However it is not clear to which extent administering such combinations can reduce glucocorticoid doses.

CA treatment including glucocorticoid treatment should be a long process lasting at least for 2 two years. Visual impairment in the context of this disease constitutes an extreme case of emergency and needs immediate therapeutic intervention (28).

12.2
Complications druing the Course of Treatment

Despite all the knowledge about the overwhelming beneficial effects of corticosteroid treatment of PMR, data concerning the optimal dosage regime are lacking. Long-term corticosteroid use can be associated with various adverse events, with the induction of osteoporosis, diabetes, hypertension or infection among the worst (24). Therefore monitoring of blood sugar levels, body weight, and blood pressure in regular intervals is mandatory (29).

Supplementation of calcium, and vitamin D should be initiated with the initiation of corticosteroids, and osteodensitomety performed to estimate the respective risk and bisphosphonates should be applied, if needed (23, 30).

It is necessary to emphasize that adverse effects may outweigh the beneficial effects of corticoid treatment. A safe prednisone dose with no risk for the development of osteoporosis has not been determined yet, however a daily prednisone doses below 5 mg can be considered relatively safe. Another aspect is that osteoporosis is known to be promoted by general inflammation. Therefore the question whether corticosteroids decrease bone mass in PMR patients or even increase it by reducing the inflammatory activity should be addressed in future investigations (31). In any case, the patients should be monitored closely, including densitometry and laboratory parameters.

As PMR constitutes a disease preferentially affecting the elderly the risk of developing diabetes mellitus in this population is obviously increased compared to younger people. It is regarded one of the main risks of prolonged corticosteroid therapy to eventually promote the development of diabetes, despite the fact that only a few clinical data concerning the likelihood of promoting diabetes by corticosteroids are existing (29). Therefore a serious risk-evaluation in PMR patients is of high interest as it might be corticosteroid dose dependent or influenced by the duration of therapy.

In addition to the risk of promoting diabetes mellitus and osteoporosis, blood pressure increase, a higher risk of infections, the worsening of a cataract and also muscle weakness can be considered other important undesirable adverse events due to corticosteroids (32). All those side effects due to the application of corticosteroids are well known, however, in the literature, not much information about the prevalence of these adverse events could be found.

Table 9   The Stockerau Corticosteroid Side Effect Questionnaire (SCSEQ) (33)

1. Do you think that the new drug alters your mood?   Yes   No
2. Do you feel depressed?   Yes   No
3. Do you think to have more infections, like common colds, since you take the new drug?   Yes   No
4. Did your body weight increase?   Yes   No
5. Do you need higher doses of anti-hypertensive drugs than before taking the new drug?   Yes   No
6. Do you suffer from alterations of the skin?   Yes   No
7. Do you suffer from muscle-weakness?   Yes   No
8. Do you suffer from alterations of the menstruation cycle?   Yes   No

Aside the objective risks of corticoid therapy some other unpleasant side effects may interfere with the patients' well being. To quantify this primarily subjective side effects a questionnaire – the so-called SCSEQ (Stockerau Corticosteroid Side Effect Questionnaire) – consisting of 7 to 8 questions with yes or no answers, was developed (33), see Table 9. This questionnaire proved to be able to discriminate between corticosteroid-users and non-users and in addition revealed a significant relationship between the daily corticosteroid dose and number of positive answers. The patient relevant adverse effects most frequently quoted by corticosteroid users were mood change, weight gain, and muscle weakness (33).

12.3
Therapy monitoring

Despite the fact that corticosteroid therapy constitutes an established measure in the treatment of PMR, no validated response criteria had been available for PMR since Barber had described the disease in 1957 (34). The gold standard of monitoring consisted of measurement of the acute phase response and patient's global assessment (8).

The development of response criteria was the other objective of the European collaborative PMR-working group. A questionnaire consisting of clinical parameters and laboratory values was developed and approved by a consensus meeting of the participating investigators. For known difficulties in standardizing clinical evaluation muscle tenderness was chosen as the only investigator dependent procedure. Laboratory examinations were performed locally according to the local standards and quality control regulations (8).

Table 10   EULAR Response Criteria for PMR (8)

1. VAS patient's pain
2. CRP or ESR
3. Morning stiffness
4. Elevation of upper limbs (0 – 3) (0 = none, 1 = below shoulder girdle, 2 = up to shoulder girdle, 3 = above shoulder girdle).
5. VAS physician's global assessment
VAS pain + three performing best of No. 2 – 5; **20%, 50%, 70%, 90% change from the baseline observation**

Seventy-six patients from all over Europe were included into this survey (69 female and 7 male patients). The observation period lasted for 48 weeks. In addition, another 24 patients recruited from the Centre for Rheumatology, Lower-Austria, was assessed according to the same protocol (8).

Patients were treated exclusively by corticosteroids; the starting dose was at the discretion of the local investigator. As a result the survey showed the expected, rapid and sustained response to glucocorticoid therapy. The daily dose could be significantly reduced throughout the study. Along with the reduction of corticosteroids nearly all parameters of disease activity, showed highly significant improvement indicating decrease of inflammatory activity, reduction of pain and amelioration of functional status of the patients (8).

Subsequently, a core set of parameters, the EULAR response criteria for PMR, was elaborated comprising the ESR or CRP, representing the acute phase response, and the VAS (visual analogue scale) of patient's pain, Physician's global assessment (PhGA), morning stiffness (MST) and the ability to elevate the upper limbs, representing the clinical situation (8).

In view of the crucial role pain plays during the course of the disease, it was decided to insist on the presence of a change of pain intensity, whereas out of the other four parameters only three have to change to indicate improvement or worsening of the disease, see Table 10. Thus to achieve a 20% response rate, and a one of 50%, 70%, 90% respectively, an amelioration of the VAS pain and three of the other four parameters is mandatory, whereby the lowest percentage change of one of the four parameters constitutes the threshold (8).

Regression and correlation analysis revealed that every single parameter of the core set is significantly influencing the individual response rate with the highest weight for VAS pain, followed by physician's assessment, CRP levels and MST and the elevation of the upper limbs, showing the lowest degree of influence on the response rate. Applying these response-criteria 50% of the patients showed a 90% improvement in week 24, the 70% response rate was at 76, 8% (8).

Monitoring disease activity in daily practice and its documentation needs to be easy to perform and not time consuming. Moreover, it should provide the physician with enough information to enable decision-making in treatment (35).

Table 11 Polymyalgia Rheumatica Disease Activity Score (PMR-AS) (12, 38)

CRP (mg/dl) + VAS pat's pain (0–10) + VAS ph ass (0–10) + [MST (min)*0,1] + Elevation of upper limbs (EUL; 3–0)') = PMR-AS (0 = above shoulder girdle, 1 = up to shoulder girdle, 2 = below shoulder girdle, 3 = none).
• remission (proposal) <1.5
• low disease activity < 7
• medium disease activity 7 – 17
• high disease activity >17

As criteria based on percentage changes from baseline may cause difficulties in daily practice, which is well known for the ACR response criteria for Rheumatoid Arthritis (36), it was considered useful to develop a simple disease activity index for PMR. Such an index, reflecting disease activity with an absolute number, would provide advantages with respect to comparability of patients and the lack of the need for of a baseline observation to assess the patient's disease actual activity [8].

Based on the core set of parameters of the PMR response criteria the disease activity index for PMR, the PMR-AS, was developed applying an easy to calculate formula:

CRP (mg/dl) * MST (min) * 0, 1 + possibility of elevation of the upper limbs (3 = none, 2 = below shoulder girdle, 1 = up to shoulder girdle, 0 = over shoulder girdle) + VAS patient's pain (0–10 cm) + VAS physician's assessment (0–10) = PMR-AS, see Table 11.

Cronbach's alpha, as a marker for reliability for composite scores amounted to 0,914 and 0,881 in two patient cohorts, indicating high internal consistency. For individual analyses a value >0.8 is regarded sufficiently valid (37). Factor analysis by principal component analysis revealed that each single item of the PMR-AS contributes significantly to the total score. Moreover the relative weight of the single items in both patient cohorts – the Pan-European and the Austrian one – was seen to be equally distributed. To evaluate whether the PMR-AS corresponds to ESR and patient's global assessment – hitherto the gold standard of monitoring PMR-patients – a third independent patient cohort was assessed. A highly significant relationship of the new composite index and those parameters could be proven (p < 0,001) (12).

Additionally a comparison of responses calculated on the basis of the PMR response criteria and the PMR-AS applied and gave congruent results. PMR-AS values below 7 can be regarded as indicating low disease activity, between 7 and 17 medium disease activity, and greater than 17 high PMR-activity (12). As a further development, it was possible to define a value <1.5 as the threshold for a remission-like state of PMR using patient relevant parameters such as pain assessment and satisfaction with disease status as bench-marks (38).

Meanwhile studies support the validity of PMR-AS in primary care practice and provides evidences that a good scoring system can be useful to guide clinical and therapeutic decisions. In addition, there is new evidence that the PMR-AS is useful for monitoring PMR activity in everyday practice and for managing glucocorticoid tapering. In this respect, PMR activity changes as expressed by the PMR-AS, seem even more relevant than absolute values (39, 40).

Thus the PMR-AS provides an easily applicable and valid tool for disease activity monitoring in patients with PMR either in clinical trials or in daily routine as it also proved to mirror patients' satisfaction with disease status (38). If used in combination with the EULAR PMR response criteria a better description of response in the evaluation of new therapies will be possible (12).

12.4
Conclusion

Polymyalgia rheumatica and giant cell arteritis are related diseases with systemic as well as local manifestations (28). Delayed diagnostics and treatment may be of serious and even lethal consequences for a patient. Arteritis of cerebral or extremity vessels resulting in stenosis or occlusion and aortic arteritis may result in dissection or rupture, especially in elderly patients. Early diagnosis of the disease, appropriate treatment and life-long monitoring of GCA patients may prevent serious complications, such as loss of vision, myocardial infarction, dissecting aortic aneurysm or critical lower-extremity ischemia and amputation. Moreover, it is important to emphasize that PMR and GCA may also occur in younger patients and with only slightly elevated inflammatory reactants and varying disease localizations (22, 28).

Given the positive treatment opportunities and excellent prognosis of the diseases on the one hand and the possible differerential diagnoses on the other there is not any room for diagnostic nihilism. Making the diagnosis of PMR/GCA with subsequent treatment commonly means rapid and dramatic improvement of the patients' complaints. As with many other diseases the only prerequisite is just to consider the possibility that PMR/GCA could be present.

References

1. Bruce W. Senile rheumatic gout. Br Med J 1888; 2: 811–813.
2. Bird HA, Esselinckx W, Dixon AS et al. An evaluation of criteria for polymyalgia rheumatica. Ann Rheum Dis 1979; 38: 434–439.
3. Jones JG, Hazleman BL. Prognosis and management of polymyalgia rheumatica. Ann Rheum Dis 1981; 40: 1–5.
4. Chuang TY, Hunder GC, Ilstrup TM, Kurland LT. Polymyalgia rheumatica: a 10-year epidemiologic and clinical study. Ann Intern Med. 1982 Nov; 97 (5): 672–80.
5. Wilke WS, Wysenbeek AJ, Krall PL et al. Masked presentation of giant-cell arteritis. Cleve Clin Q 1985; 52 (2): 155–159.
6. Nobunaga M, Yoshioka K, Yasuda M et al. Clinical studies of polymyalgia rheumatica: a proposal of diagnostic criteria. Jpn J Med 1989; 28 (4): 452–456.

12

7. Bird HA, Leeb BF, Montecucco CM et al. A comparison of the sensitivity of diagnostic criteria for polymyalgia rheumatica. Ann Rheum Dis 2005; 64 (4): 626–629.

8. Leeb BF, Bird HA, Nesher G et al. EULAR response criteria for polymyalgia rheumatica. Results of an initiative of the European collaborating Polymyalgia Rheumatica group (Subcommittee of ESCISIT [EULAR Standing Committee on Clinical Trials Including Therapeutical Trials]); Ann Rheum Dis 2003; 62: 1189–1194.

9. Hunder GG, Bloch DA, Michel BA et al. The American College of Rheumatology 1990 criteria for the classification of giant cell arteritis. Arthritis Rheum 1990; 33 (8): 1122–1128.

10. Nothnagl T, Leeb BF. Diagnosis, differential diagnosis and treatment of polymyalgia rheumatica. Drugs Aging 2006; 23 (5): 391–402.

11. Hunder GG. Giant cell arteritis and polymyalgia rheumatica. Med Clin North Amer 1997; 81: 195–219.

12. Leeb BF, Bird HA. A disease activity score for polymyalgia rheumatica – PMR-AS. Ann Rheum Dis 2004; 63: 1279–1283.

13. Pease CT, Haugeberg G, Montague B, Hensor EM, Bhakta BB, Thomson W, Ollier WE, Morgan AW. Polymyalgia rheumatica can be distinguished from late onset rheumatoid arthritis at baseline: results of a 5-yr prospective study. Rheumatol (Oxford) 2009 Feb; 48 (2): 123–7. Epub 2008 Nov 2

14. De Silva M, Hazleman BL. Azathioprine in giant cell arteritis/polymyalgia rheumatica: a double-blind study. Ann Rheum Dis 1986; 45 (2): 136–138.

15. Feinberg HL, Shennan JD, Schrepferman CG et al. The use of methotrexate in polymyalgia rheumatica. J Rheumatol 1996; 23 (9): 1550–1552.

16. Ferraccioli G, Salaffi F, De Vita S et al. Methotrexate in polymyalgia rheumatica: preliminary results of an open, ran-domized study. Rheumatol 1996; 23 (4): 624–628.

17. Salvarani C, Cantini F, Niccoli L et al. Treatment of refractory polymyalgia rheumatica with infliximab: a pilot study. J Rheumatol 2003; 30 (4): 760–763.

18. Tan AL, Holdsworth J, Pease C et al. Successful treatment of resistant giant cell arteritis with etanercept. Ann Rheum Dis 2003; 62: 373–374.

19. Hoffman GS, Cid MC, Rendt-Zagar KE, Merkel PA, Weyand CM, Stone JH, Salvarani C, Xu W, Visvanathan S, Rahman MU. Infliximab-GCA Study Group Infliximab for maintenance of glucocorticosteroid-induced remission of giant cell arteritis: a randomized trial. Ann Intern Med. 2007 May 1; 146 (9): 621–30.

20. Martínez-Taboada VM, Rodríguez-Valverde V, Carreño L, López-Longo J, Figueroa M, Belzunegui J, Mola EM, Bonilla G. A double-blind placebo controlled trial of etanercept in patients with giant cell arteritis and corticosteroid side effects. Ann Rheum Dis 2008 May; 67 (5): 625–30. Epub 2007 Dec 17

21. Straub RH, Gluck T, Cutolo M et al. The adrenal steroid status in relation to inflammatory cytokines (interleukin-6 and tumour necrosis factor) in polymyalgia rheumatica. Rheumatol (Oxford) 2000; 39: 624–631.

22. Proven A, Gabriel SE, O'Fallon WM et al. Polymyalgia rheumatica with low erythrocyte sedimentation rate at diagnosis. J Rheumatol 1999; 26: 1333–1337.

23. Pavelka K. Polymyalgia rheumatica a temporální arteriitida. Čes Revmatol 2001; 9 (3): 129–136 (in Czech).

24. Gabriel SE, Sunku J, Salvarani C et al. Adverse outcomes of antiinflammatory therapy among patients with polymyalgia rheumatica. Arthritis Rheum 1997; 40 (10): 1873–1878.

25. De Silva M, Hazleman BL. Azathioprine in giant cell arteritis/polymyalgia rheumatica: a double-blind study. Ann Rheum Dis 1986; 45 (2): 136–138.

26. Feinberg HL, Shennan JD, Schrepferman CG et al. The use of methotrexate in polymyalgia rheumatica. J Rheumatol 1996; 23 (9): 1550–1552.

27. Ferraccioli G, Salaffi F, De Vita S et al. Methotrexate in polymyalgia rheumatica: preliminary results of an open, ran-domized study. Rheumatol 1996; 23 (4): 624–628.

28. Salvarani C, Cantini F, Boiardi L et al. Polymyalgia rheumatica and giant cell arteritis. N Engl J Med 2002; 347: 261–271.

29.   Panthakalam S, Bhatnagar D, Klimiuk P. The prevalence and management of hypergly-caemia in patients with rheumatoid arthritis on corticosteroid therapy. Scott Med J 2004; 49 (4): 139–141.

30.   Woolf AD. An update on glucocorticoid-induced osteoporosis. Curr Opin Rheumatol 2007 Jul; 19 (4): 370–375.

31.   Lodder MC, de Jong Z, Kostense PJ et al. Bone mineral density in patients with rheumatoid arthritis: relation between disease severity and low bone mineral density. Ann Rheum Dis 2004; 63 (12): 1576–1580 Long-term follow-up of polymyalgia rheumatica patients treated with methotrexate and steroids.

32.   Cimmino MA, Salvarani C, Macchioni P, Gerli R, Bartoloni Bocci E, Montecucco C, Caporali R. Systemic Vasculitis Study Group of the Italian Society for Rheumatology. Long-term follow-up of polymyalgia rheumatica patients treated with methotrexate and steroids. Clin Exp Rheumatol 2008 May/Jun; 26 (3): 395–400.

33.   Svoboda T, Andel I, Burgschmidt I et al. A corticosteroid side effect questionnaire discriminates between corticosteroid using and not-using patients with rheumatoid arthritis (RA) and polymyalgia rheumatica (PMR). Ann Rheum Dis 2004 Suppl. I: 174 (THU 0221); EULAR 2004, Berlin.

34.   Barber HS. Myalgic syndrome with constitutional effects; polymyalgia rheumatica. Ann Rheum Dis 1957 Jun; 16 (2): 230–237.

35.   Furst DE, Breedveld FC, Kalden JR, Smolen JS, Antoni CE, Bijlsma JW et al. Updated consensus statement on biological agents for the treatment of rheumatoid arthritis and other rheumatic diseases (May 2002). Ann Rheum Dis 2001; 61 (Suppl II) ii2–ii7.

36.   Felson DT, Anderson JJ, Boers M, Bombardier C, Chernoff M, Fried B, et al. The American College of Rheumatology Preliminary Core Set of Disease Activity Measures for Rheumatoid Arthritis Clinical Trials. Arthritis Rheum 1993; 36: 729–740.

37.   Streiner DL. Starting at the beginning: An introduction to coefficient alpha and internal consistency. J Pers Assess 2003; 80 (1): 99–103.

38.   Leeb BF, Rintelen B, Sautner J, Fassl Ch, Bird HA. The Polymyalgia Rheumatica Activity Score (PMR-AS) in daily use – Proposal for a definition of remission. Arthritis Rheum 2007 Jun 15; 57 (5): 810–815. 2007.

39.   Binard A, Lefebvre B, De Bandt M, Berthelot JM, Saraux A. Club "Rhumatismes et Inflammation": Validity of the Polymyalgia Rheumatica Activity Score in primary care practice. Ann Rheum Dis 2009 Apr; 68 (4): 541–545. Epub 2008 May 13

40.   Binard A, de Bandt M, Berthelot JM, Saraux A. Inflammatory Joint Disease Working Group of the French Society for Rheumatology. Performance of the polymyalgia rheumatica activity score for diagnosing disease flares. Arthritis Rheum 2008 Feb 15; 59 (2): 263–269.

Figures

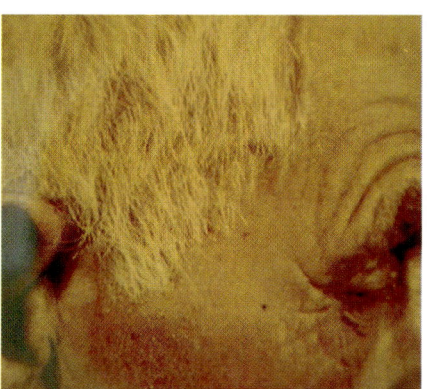

Fig. 1
Patient with temporal arteritis.

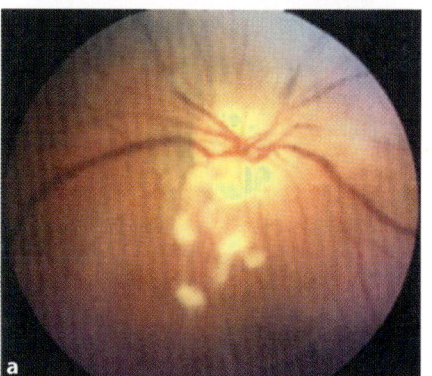

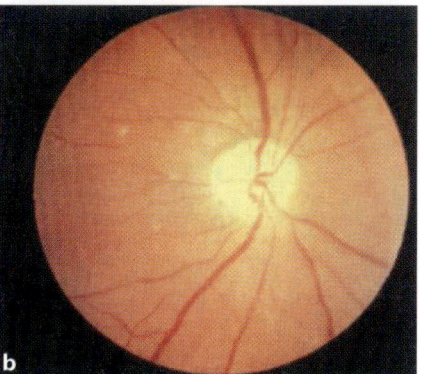

Fig. 2
a, b Loss of vision is a serious complication. The slide shows ischemic alterations of the ocular nerve disk and the retina of the right eye prior to glucocorticoids therapy; in the next picture we can see improvement in the right eye fundus after administration of gluco-corticoids. Administration of high doses of steroids can save the patient's vision.

Fig. 3
Impaired convergence and ptosis of
the upper left lid. Temporal arteritis
presenting with paresis of the oculomotor nerve and PMR, despite
a low ESR.

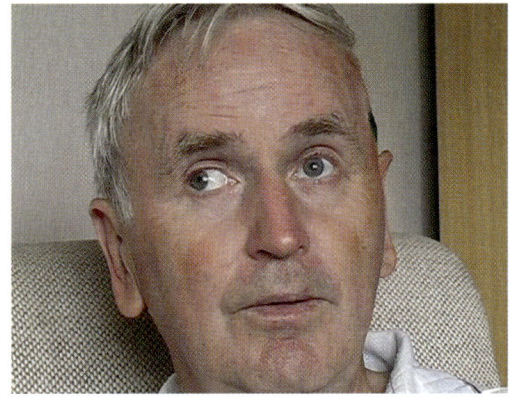

Fig. 4
a, **b** Fatal outcome of PMR/GCA, histologically
confirmed arteritis of the peripheral vessels of the
lower extremities, with subsequent gangrene and
amputation of the right lower extremity and gangrene on the left big toe and the second toe. Later,
after the amputation of left toes, pulmonary artery
embolism occured.

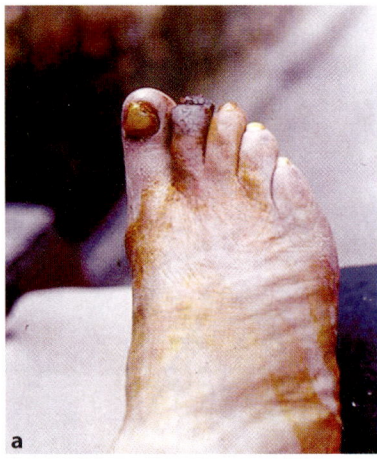

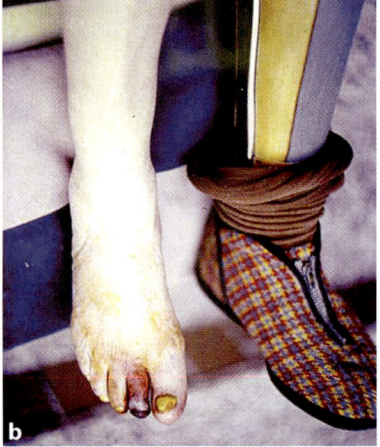

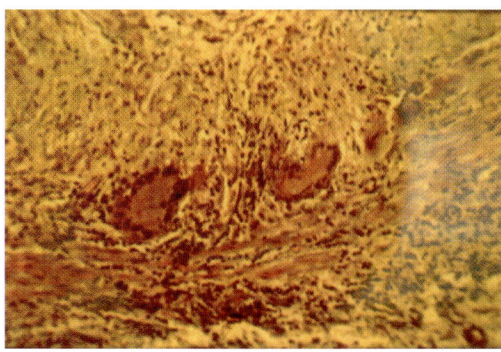

Fig. 5
Giant cell arteritis with Horton cells.

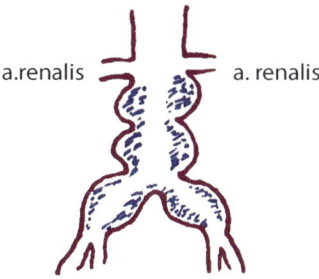

a.renalis   a. renalis

Fig. 6
Scheme of the aneurysms of abdominal aorta and common iliac arteries in an 86 year old man.

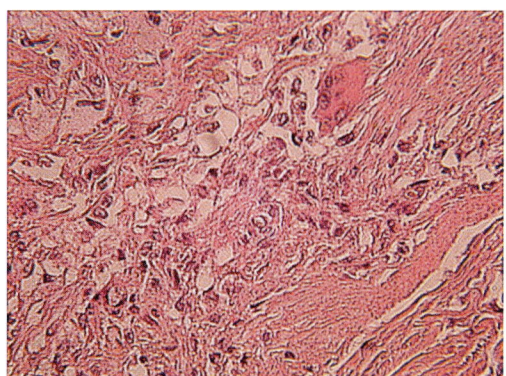

Fig. 7
Granulomatous inflammation of the media of abdominal aorta. Stained with HE – hematoxylin – eosin. Inflammatory infiltration formed mainly by histiocytes and plasmatic cells, less from lymphocytes, multinucleated giant cells.

Fig. 8
Multinucleated giant cell. Stained
with HE.

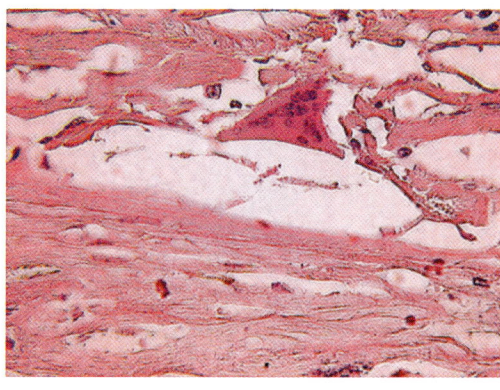

Fig. 9
Dissected and fragmentated lamina
elastica interna. Stained with HE.

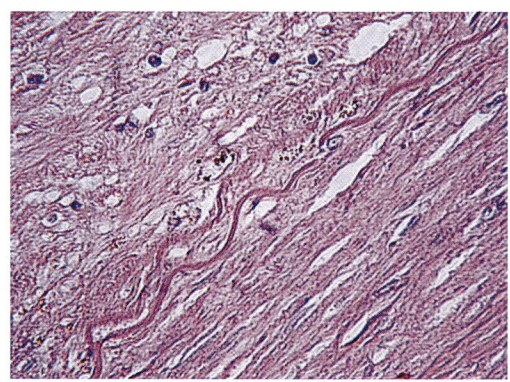

Fig. 10
Multinucleated giant cells. Stained
with HE.

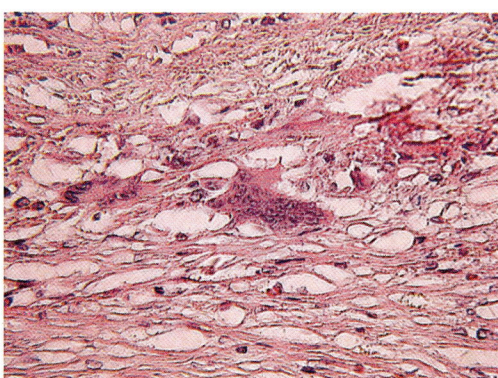

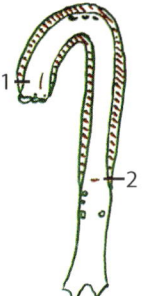

Fig. 11
Scheme of dissecting aneurysm of
the thoracic and abdominal aorta in
an 84 year old woman. 1 – beginning
of the dissection, 2 – end of the dissection.

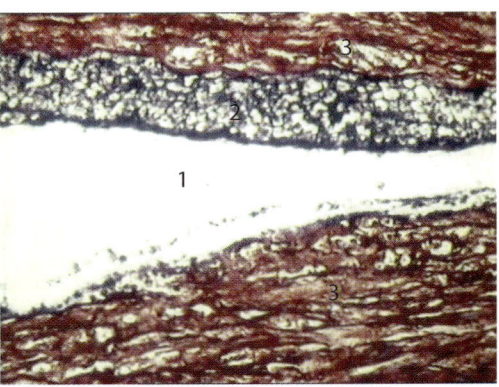

Fig. 12
Dissecting aneurysm of aorta in
a patient with giant cells arteritis –
dissection (1), fibrin (2), and media
(3). Stained with fosfowolfram hematoxylin.

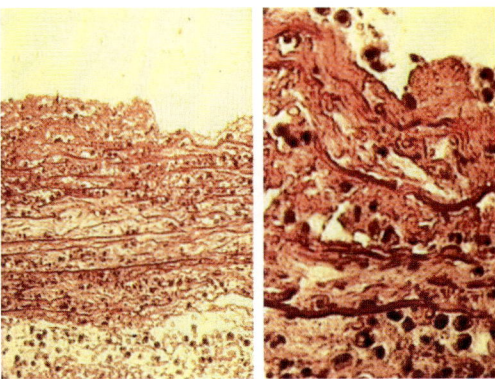

Fig. 13   Panarteritis – mixed inflammatory infiltrate. Stained with hematoxylin – eosin (HE).

Fig. 14
Calcium deposits (1) in lamina
elastica interna, sclerotic plaque
with calcium in intima (2). Stained
with Kossa and HE.

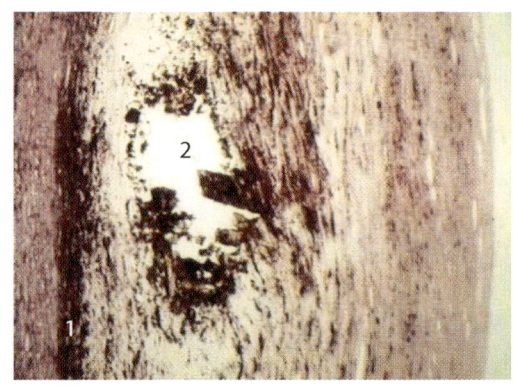

Fig. 15
Typical calcium powder in lamina
elastica interna (l.e.i). Stained with
Kossa and HE.

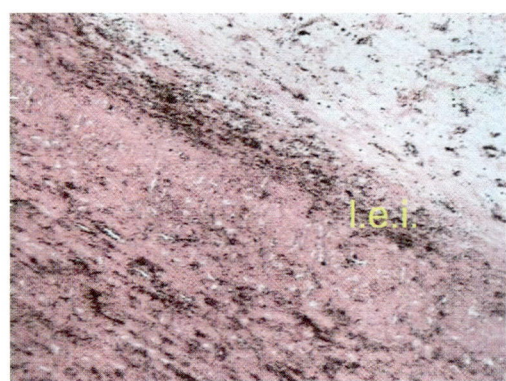

Fig. 16
Macroscopic photography of the
aortic arch – dissection of the aortic
wall with blood coagulum.

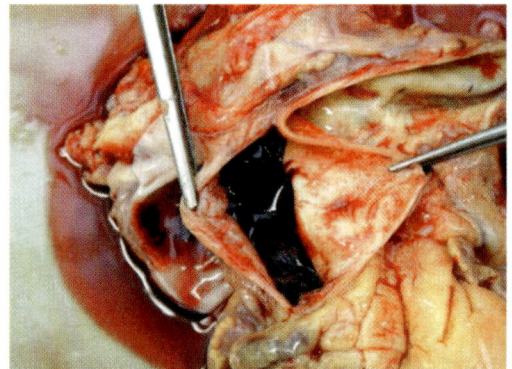

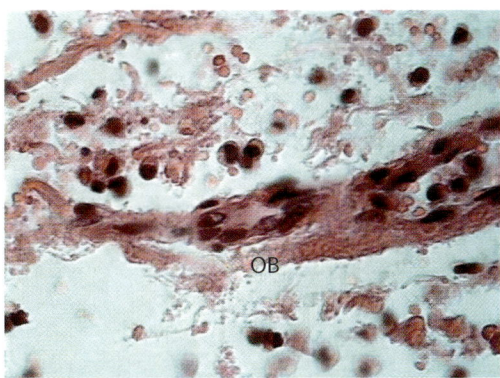

Fig. 17
Aortic wall – mixed inflammatory
infiltrate, histiocytes and giant cell
(OB) in adventitia. Stained with HE.

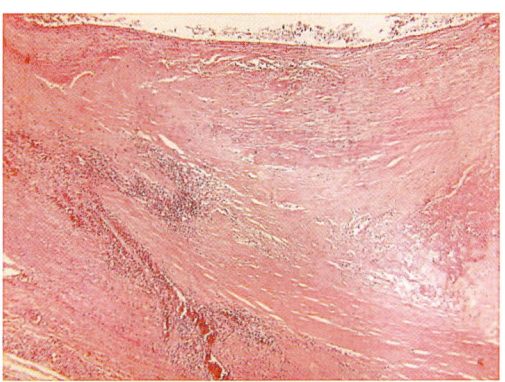

Fig. 18
Neovascularisation in the media of
aorta.

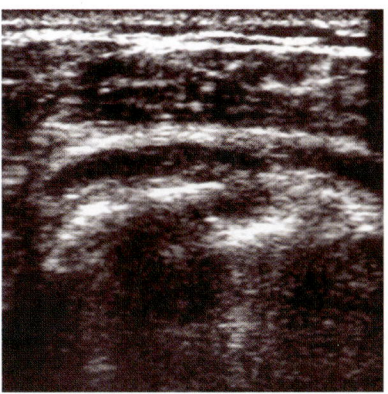

Fig. 19
Image of the right shoulder, small
amount of fluid in the subdeltoid
bursa and in the intraarticular space.

Fig. 20
Ultrasonographic image of the left hip joint, dilatation of capsule with small amount of fluid in the intraarticular space.

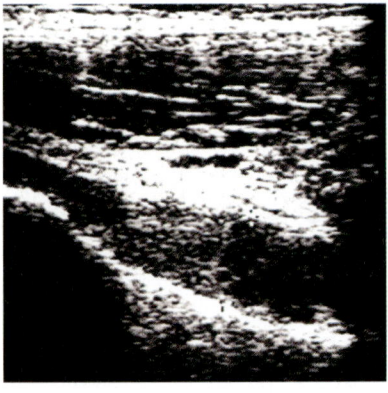

Fig. 21
Color duplex image of temporal artery, longitudinal section with hypoechogenic edematous arterial wall in patient with TA.

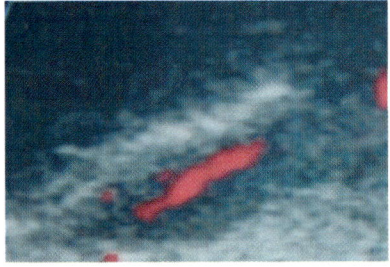

Fig. 22
Color duplex image of temporal artery, transversal section of edematous wall with "halo" effect in patient with active TA.

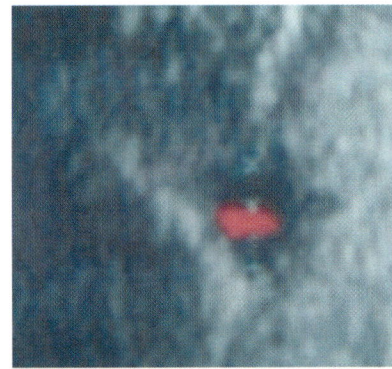

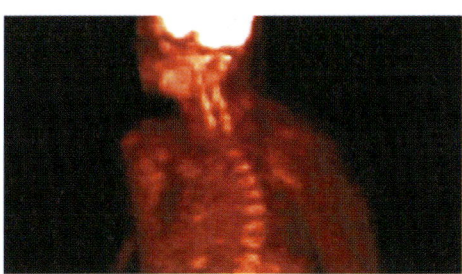

Fig. 23
In PET/18FDG examination, symmetrically increased 18FDG metabolisation in
the neck area occurs in both carotids.

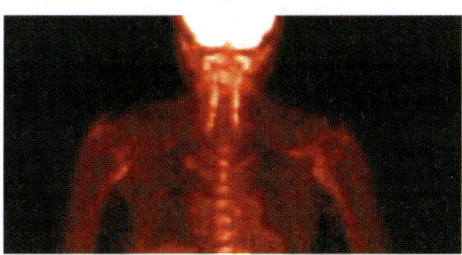

Fig. 24
Symmetrically increased 18FD cumula-
tions along carotids are visible. It may be
a confirmation of arteritis.